Intermittent Fasting for Women Over 50

3 Books in 1:

The Complete Collection to Improve Your Health and Detox Your Body While Losing Weight and Boosting Metabolism

By

Asuka Young

Table of Contents

INTERMITTENT FASTING FOR WOMEN OVER 50

INTERMITTENT FASTING 16/8

INTERMITTENT FASTING FOR WOMEN

INTERMITTENT FASTING FOR WOMEN OVER 50

The Ultimate Guide For Senior Women To Promote Longevity While Losing Weight & Increase Energy Through Metabolic Autophagy

By

Asuka Young

Introduction

Fasting intermittently is not a diet. It's an eating habit and a lifestyle. It's a way to prepare the meals to ensure that one gets the best out of them. Fasting Intermittently doesn't affect what you consume. It matters when you consume food. Intermittent fasting is not only a method for weight reduction or a hack that athletes use to lose fat while easily keeping lean muscle mass. It is a balanced lifestyle influenced by human evolution and the research on metabolism at its finest. Intermittent fasting needs the body to be more self-productive and effective for it to work. Intermittent fasting typically implies that, you intake the calories at a specific time and choose not to eat food for a longer time. Many research indicates that this form of living can provide benefits such as weight reduction, improved fitness, and enhanced lifespan. Experts claim that it's simpler to sustain an extended fasting regimen than conventional, calorie-controlled diets. Understanding the intermittent fasting of each person is different, and varying types will fit other individuals based on their needs.

Fasting intermittently is one of the best methods people have for reducing excess weight off but holding healthy weight on, and it needs relatively least behavior modification. This is a positive idea because it ensures intermittent fasting fits under the easy enough task that one will simply do it, however significant enough that it can make a transformation. Intermittent fasting shifts hormone levels to promote weight reduction.

In addition to reducing insulin in the bloodstream and increasing growth hormone levels, it enhances the production of the burning fat hormone known as noradrenaline or norepinephrine.

Studies suggest that a very effective method for weight reduction may be intermittent fasting. Short-term fasting can raise the body's metabolic rate by 3.6 to 14 percent due to these hormones' changes. By encouraging one to eat less, burn additional calories, by manipulating all calorie calculation aspects, intermittent fasting induces weight loss.

In contrast to other weight loss trials, a review study showed that this eating style would induce 3 to 8 percent weight loss from 3 to 24 weeks, which is a significant change. There is no each-size-fits-all approach when it comes to intermittent fasting at the end of the day. The one approach that you should hold on to in the long term is the right pattern with proper nutrition for you.

For certain individuals, intermittent fasting is fine, just not for others. Although, in particular, older people over 50 and women may try it comfortably. Trying it out is the best way to figure out which group you relate to. It can be an effective method to lose weight and boost your wellbeing if you feel comfortable while fasting and believe it to be a sustainable form of eating.

Chapter 1:
What is Intermittent Fasting

During intermittent fasting, you would not be pressured to deprive yourself throughout the day, also mentioned as IF. It also doesn't grant you a license during the period of non-fasting to eat loads of unhealthy food. You consume within a fixed window of time, instead of consuming meals and treats all day. Intermittent fasting is an eating pattern model that requires daily, short-term fasts or limited or no food intake at times.

Most individuals know intermittent fasting as losing weight assistance. Intermittent fasting is a lifestyle that allows people to consume fewer calories, leading to weight loss over time.

Without being on an insane diet or consuming the calories to nil, it's a perfect way to get healthy. Most of the time, when one begins intermittent fasting, they'll aim to maintain their calories the same as during a shortened time; most people consume larger meals. In comparison, prolonged fasting is a healthy way to preserve body mass while becoming lean. But most notably, intermittent fasting is among the most beneficial way to be in shape with many other benefits. This is an easy way to get the desired results. If performed properly, intermittent fasting will have valuable advantages, like weight reduction, type 2 diabetes reversal, and several other aspects. Plus, this will save time and resources for you.

Intermittent fasting is successful because it makes it possible for the amount of insulin and blood sugar to reach a low level. The body's fat-storing enzyme is insulin. Fat moves into the fat cells and gets absorbed when insulin levels are high in the blood; if insulin level is low, fat will move and burn out of fat cells. In short, IF is when food is readily available, but you prefer not to consume it. This may be over any period of time, from several hours to a couple of days, or sometimes a week or more under strict medical monitoring. You can begin fasting at any moment of your choice, and you can end a fast at your will, too.

You fast intermittently if you don't consume food by choice. For instance, between dinner and breakfast, till the following day, you will not eat and fast for around 12 to 14 hours. Intermittent fasting can, in that way, be deemed a part of daily life.

1.1 How Intermittent Fasting works

There are many intermittent fasting methods, but all of them are focused on consuming a diet over daily time periods. For instance, every day, a person can try to eat only during a nine-hour cycle and fast for the rest. Or 2 days a week, you could want to eat just one meal a day. Several intermittent fasting routines are different.

The metabolic switching state refers to the body exhausting its sugar reserves after hours without consuming any calories and beginning to burn fat. On the molecular and cellular scale, when a person fasts, many things happen in the body. The body changes hormone levels, for example, to make retained body fat more available. Intermittent fasting works in stages.

1.2 Stages of Intermittent Fasting

- After 12 hours of fasting, the body has reached the metabolic stage of ketosis. The body continues to burn and break down fat in this condition.

- After 18 hours, the body has moved to the fat-burning mode and produces essential ketones.

- After 24 hours, the body's cells are gradually replacing old components and breaking down defected proteins associated with Alzheimer's and other neurodegenerative diseases. This is a strategy called autophagy.

For tissue and cell rejuvenation, autophagy is an essential mechanism that eliminates weakened cellular components, including defected proteins. Severe consequences happen when the cells don't or can't activate autophagy, like many neurodegenerative disorders, which tend to develop due to the diminished autophagy during aging.

- After 48 hours, the body's growth hormone output is up by five times as strong, without consuming calories or with very little calories, carbohydrates, or protein when one began their fast.

This process explains that ketone bodies formed throughout fasting can facilitate growth hormone secretion in the brain. Ghrelin, the starvation hormone, often promote development hormone secretion. Growth hormone helps maintain lean muscle mass, particularly as we mature, and it decreases the buildup of fat tissue. It also tends to play a part in humans' survival and may facilitate cardiovascular wellbeing and wound healing.

- After 54 hours,' insulin has fallen to its lowest amount after a person has begun fasting, and the body gets more and more insulin-sensitive. Decreased amounts of insulin provide a variety of long-term and short-term health effects.

- After 72 hours, the body breaks down aged immune cells and creates new ones.

- Intermittent fasting can also influence risk factors, such as blood sugar levels and reducing cholesterol, for health problems such as cardiovascular disease and diabetes.

During fasting, Important repair mechanisms are often performed by the cells which alter the expression of genes. One can lose weight with intermittent fasting, as it also impacts the hormones. It's because it is the way, body processes body fat as energy calories. The body makes many improvements when you do not consume something and allow the accumulated energy more usable.

Examples involve shifts in the nervous system's function and drastic changes in certain essential hormones' quantities.

Two metabolic modifications mentioned below that occur when a person fast

- Insulin: When a person consumes food, insulin levels rise, and when fasting began, they decline drastically. Fat burning is encouraged by reduced amounts of insulin.

- Norepinephrine or Noradrenaline: Norepinephrine is forwarded to the fat cells by the nervous system, allowing them to disintegrate body fat into unsaturated fatty acids that can be used for energy.

Here are several alterations that occur while fasting in the human body:

- (HGH)Human Growth Hormone: Growth hormone levels rise exponentially, by as many as five times. This has muscle gain and fat loss advantages as well as many others.

- Insulin: Sensitivity to insulin increases, and insulin levels decrease significantly. Low levels of insulin improve the ability of the body to use stored fat.

- Cellular repair: The cells begin cellular repair while fasting. This means autophagy, where aged and damaged proteins build up within cells, digest, and kill unhealthy cells.

- Gene expression: There are improvements in longevity-related gene expression and defense against disease.

Intermittent fasting's health benefits can be seen as these variations in hormone levels, cell structure, and gene expression occur.

Chapter 2:
Intermittent Fasting for Women Over 50

According to researchers, intermittent fasting is beneficial for most people who eat during their daytime hours. Prolonged fasting differs from the usual eating style. If someone consumes 3 meals per day, including treats, and they don't work out, they operate on certain calories and don't burn their fat reserves at any time. Intermittent fasting allows our bodies to burn the reserved fat storage in a healthy way; nine older women in ten have a form of chronic illness, and nearly eight in ten have more than one chronic disease. So, odds are, eventually, a person will get more. But to live a healthy life, there are measures one should take, and fasting intermittently is one of them.

Many of these chronic illnesses start from being overweight at an older age. The most important aspect of intermittent fasting is its weight loss assistance. Another research found that intermittent fasting induces less muscle loss than the more traditional form of daily restriction of calories. Bear in mind, though, that the primary explanation for its effectiveness is that intermittent fasting allows you to intake fewer calories overall. During your meal times, if you indulge and consume large quantities, you will not lose much weight at all.

2.1 Why Start Intermittent Fasting After 50?

Here, excess weight in women can cause these diseases, and intermittent fasting can help counteract them. Furthermore, intermittent fasting can help you control these aspects of living if you are over 50.

- Hypertension

With age, blood vessels become less elastic when a person' matures. This puts a strain on the mechanism that holds the body's blood. It may indicate why 2 in 3 women over the age of 50 have elevated blood pressure. The best approach to manage hypertension is to lose weight by intermittent fasting.

- Diabetes

At least one in 10 women has diabetes. When you grow older, the odds of having the disease increase up. Heart failure, renal disease, blindness, and other complications may arise from diabetes due to excess weight.

- Cardiac Condition

A significant source of heart attack is plaque formation in the arteries due to unhealthy eating. It begins in youth, and as one matures, it becomes worse. A large percentage of men and 5.6 percent of women have suffered from heart failure in the 40-58 age range in the U.S. Fasting and eating healthy is a good option to control any cardiovascular diseases

- Obesity

It might be dangerous for the health if one weighs too much for their height; it's not about getting a few extra pounds. More than 20 obesity chronic illnesses are correlated with stroke, asthma, arthritis, cancer, coronary failure, and high blood pressure. At least 30% of the older population is obese.

- Arthritis

This condition of the joints was once directly attributed by physicians to the excessive wear and tear of time, and it sure is a cause. Yet biology and lifestyle are likely to have still much to do with it. A lack of physical exercise, diabetes, and becoming overweight may play a role in past joint accidents, too.

- Osteoporosis

With old age, bones become weak, especially in women, which may lead to fractures. It impacts nearly 53.9 million Americans over 50 years of age. A few factors that will help: a balanced diet high in vitamin D and Calcium, losing excess weight by fasting, and daily weight-bearing activity, such as walking, jogging, and climbing stairs

- Tumor & Cancers

The greatest risk factor for old age is cancer. The disorder also impacts young adults, but between the ages of 46 and 54, your risk of getting it more than doubles. You can't influence a person's age or genes, but you have a choice in stuff like smoking or living an unhealthy lifestyle. With much of the study focusing on the beneficial impact, fasting has on cancer, fasting over varying periods of time has often helped older women decrease their risk of severe diseases. The study reported that fasting appears to suppress some cancer-causing pathways and can even delay tumor development.

- Menopause

The classic indicators of menopause are hot flashes, insomnia, night sweats, mood swings, vaginal dryness, burning, and itching. Heart failure and osteoporosis appear to escalate throughout the years of menopause. Often people start prolonged fasting to combat both the long-term and short-term symptoms of menopause. For several post-menopausal women, Belly fat, not just for appearance but also for health, is a major concern. The decrease in belly fat resulting from intermittent fasting helped women minimize their likelihood of metabolic syndrome, a series of health conditions that enhance the risk of heart disease and diabetes for a post-menopausal female.

2.2 Advantages of Intermittent Fasting for Women Over 50

The benefits of intermittent fasting for women over 50 are limitless; some of them are mentioned here:

- Decrease of insulin resistance, Fasting is one of the most successful strategies to return the insulin receptors to a normal sensitivity level. Understanding the function of insulin plays is one of the biggest keys to learning about fasting and truly understanding every diet. In relation to eating, insulin, the hormone that controls blood sugar, is formed in the pancreas and absorbed into the bloodstream. Insulin allows the body to retain energy as fat until released. Insulin creates fat because the fatter the body stores, the more insulin body makes or vice versa. The cycles during which a person is not eating allow the body time to reduce insulin levels, mainly during intermittent fasting, which changes the fat-storing mechanism. The mechanism goes in reverse, and the body loses weight as insulin levels decrease.

- Autophagy is the incredible way the cells "eat themselves" in order to get rid of dead cells and recycle the younger parts. Autophagy is often the mechanism by which harmful pathogens, including viruses, bacteria, and other diseases, are killed. As the whole cell is recycled, another step in apoptosis. Your chance of cancer rises without this process when defective cells tend to multiply.

- Intermittent fasting leads to Detoxification. Many of us have been subjected to contaminants from food and our climate in our lifetime. Many of these containments are processed in our bodies in fat cells. One of the most powerful methods to eliminate contaminants from the body is fasting and eating healthy.

- The body's internal clock or Circadian Rhythm of the body controls virtually any mechanism in the body, and a chain of detrimental results will occur when it is disturbed. You adjust the circadian clock of the body while you take a rest from meals.

- A Healthy Gut is one of the most important aspects of Fasting in that it provides a chance for the digestive tract and intestinal flora to reset. This is critical because the health of the body's digestive system regulates the immune system. There is even more proof that one's moods and emotional wellbeing are co-dependent on the gut microbiota. In recent studies of any area related to health and wellbeing, there has been a lot of hype on how one's gut flora might play an important part. The work of a more powerful immune system is important to a diverse microbiota, and it plays an important role in one's mental wellbeing. It also removes skin problems and reduces cancer danger. Although the foods you consume have an immense effect on your intestinal health, periodic fasting in the digestive system can be another way to help grow the beneficial bacteria in the gut. Sugar and artificial goods disturb the equilibrium of your digestive tract between the beneficial and detrimental microbiota. Make sure to minimize packaged foods full of refined carbohydrates, sugars, and harmful fats to get the best outcome if you try intermittent fasting. Alternatively, switch to whole grains, plenty of organic vegetables and fruits, and good quality protein.

- Intermittent fasting will work better by metabolic switching. Fasting contributes to lower glucose levels in the bloodstream. The body utilizes fat as an energy source instead of sugar after converting the fat into ketones.

- Although it's not fasting, several physicians have recorded intermittent fasting advantages by permitting some easy-to-digest foods during the fasting window as fresh fruit. Modifications like this will also provide the essential rest for your metabolic and digestive system.

- Losing weight: it is expected that fasting helps accelerate the loss of excess weight. It also decreases insulin levels such that the body no longer receives the message to store more calories as fat during the state of fasting. Intermittent fasting may contribute to a self-activating decrease in calorie consumption by letting you consume fewer meals. In addition, to promote weight reduction, prolonged fasting affects hormone levels. It enhances noradrenaline or norepinephrine production, which is a fat-burning hormone, lowering insulin and rising growth hormone levels. Intermittent fasting can increase one's metabolic rate due to these changes in hormones. By encouraging one to eat less and activating ketones' production, and by adjusting all calorie calculation factors, intermittent fasting induces weight loss. In contrast to other weight loss trials, a study showed that this eating method would cause 3-8 percent weight loss in just weeks, which is a substantial percentage. People have lost 4 to 7 percent of their waist circumference, as per the same report, it is helpful for women dealing with menopause and unhealthy stomach fat that builds up over their organs and induces illness.

Other than insulin, during intermittent fasting are two important hormones, leptin and ghrelin. Ghrelin is the hormone of starvation that tells the body when it's hungry. Research shows that ghrelin can be reduced by intermittent fasting. There is also some evidence suggesting a rise in the leptin hormone, the hormone of satiety. That tells the body when it's full, and there's no more urge to eat.

- People would be fuller quicker and hungry less frequently with less ghrelin and more leptin, which may lead to fewer calories eaten and, as a result, weight loss.

Other benefits of intermittent fasting in women over 50 are

- Alzheimer's disorder in women over 50 and other neurodegenerative diseases may be severe. There are many lifestyle options that scientists claim, including extended fasting, may help avoid Alzheimer's. Recent research released says prolonged fasting preserve the polarization of aquaporin-4 in the brain. It can help defend against Alzheimer's. Aquaporin-4 plays a key function in the elimination of amyloid-β, a peptide thought to contribute to Alzheimer's. Intermittent fasting may be one of the best approaches to lower the risk of Alzheimer's, getting a brain boost alongside a well-balanced diet and daily exercise.

- Depression & Intermittent Fasting

Personal wellbeing factors are taken into account in the evaluation research. Several findings show that women who follow distinct fasting strategies reported change in their moods for better self-esteem, reducing depression and anxiety.

- IF Increases Joint & Muscle Health

According to research, fasting increased muscle and joint protection because low back pain and arthritic symptoms were not as prominent.

- Inflammation Reduction

According to research, many women over 50 during intermittent fasting reported that they have achieved a decline in oxidative stress and inflammation, which is extremely significant, considering the vast number of women had breast cancer family history. There is also not an increase in ghrelin, the hormone of hunger, which is beneficial.

- Maintaining Metabolism

A decrease in the resting rate of metabolic or 'metabolism' is one issue that can occur with weight loss. It makes it difficult to lose weight as this happens, the body doesn't burn many calories. Still, intermittent fasting helps the metabolism rate increase so that women over 50 easily lose excess weight with fasting.

IF also Improves LDL cholesterol, total cholesterol and triglycerides, and blood pressure for the better. The same advantages are experienced by the women doing 5:2 fasting or any other way of intermittent fasting. With daily alternating fasting, both women and men can experience a substantial drop in insulin, increased ketones, and unsaturated fatty acids, meaning that women would benefit as much as men.

As a woman over 50, you can maximize intermittent fasting advantages by following these few points:

- Sugar and processed grains should be avoided. Eat apples, whole grains, vegetables, beans, lean proteins, lentils, and good fats (a good, Mediterranean-style diet based on plants).

- Between meals, let the body burn fat. Don't snack on unhealthy foods. During your day, be productive. Develop your lean muscles.

- Consider a more effective form of intermittent fasting. Restrict the day's hours to consume calories, and make it early in the day for a better effect.

- Avoid getting sweets or consuming all the time at night.

In addition, certain senior women may need to consume food daily due to their metabolic conditions or prescription guidelines; under any scenario, before making any adjustments, a person should address their dietary patterns with care practitioners.

2.3 Potential Risks of Intermittent Fasting for Women Over 50

Certainly, prolonged fasting might not be for everyone. If you are undernourished or have a record of eating disorders, you must not start intermittent fast without first speaking with a health provider. There is some proof that intermittent fasting for some women might not be as effective for men. For instance, one research found that it increased insulin sensitivity in males than females. Still, in certain women that blood sugar regulation worsens, it may be because of some women's underlying condition.

You should contact a doctor before attempting intermittent fasting if you have a medical problem. This is especially relevant for you if:

- Taking medications.
- Having diabetes
- Having problems with blood sugar regulation.
- Are underweight.
- Have a history of eating disorders
- Have a history of amenorrhea
- Have low blood pressure.

Although intermittent fasting shows potential, we don't have clear proof of the long-term impact of how often older adults might be influenced by fasting. Human experiments have mainly focused on category includes middle-aged and young people for a brief amount of time. Yet we do know that, in certain situations, intermittent fasting might be dangerous. As far as low body weight is concerned, it is worrisome that a person would lose so much weight, impacting their bones, energy level, and overall immune system.

According to doctors, People who need their medication to survive with food to prevent discomfort or stomach irritation cannot do well with intermittent fasting. People who take cardiac or blood pressure drugs may also be more likely to develop harmful sodium and potassium imbalances as they try to fast.

If you have diabetes and require food after some hours or taking medicine that influences your blood sugar, intermittent fasting can even be dangerous.

If intermittent fasting is important for wellbeing, causing you hunger pangs will interrupt sleep. It could even render you less conscious or aware. Intermittent fasting will contribute to reducing alertness since the body does not eat sufficient calories to provide enough nutrition during a fasting window. Fasting can also contribute to tiredness, problems focusing, or dizziness.

If you leave the fast too early, the diet does not entail guilt or self-shaming—a potential sign of disordered behavior, maybe some form of fear or embarrassment surrounding your fast.

While intermittent fasting is a very beneficial solution for women over 50, you can also rethink intermittent fasting if you notice these symptoms and signs:

- It could be linked to fasting if someone experiences hair loss.

- In the starting stages of intermittent fasting, thirst, exhaustion, and fatigue are very common.

- During the feeding time, overeating or not eating nutritious foods leads to extreme hunger.

- Heartburn or reflux owing to heavy eating.

A hint that intermittent fasting may not be safe for you is the feelings of fear, sadness, or anti-social emotions.

While intermittent fasting is not inherently harmful, individuals with an eating condition or family or a personal background must stay clear of the diet. For those extremely active, intermittent fasting is also not suitable because they need more energy.

Food gives our body movement energy, so exercising while fasting will impact efficiency and contribute to an unsafe energy deficiency. Focus on healthy, nutrient-packed options, such as fruits, veggies, lean meats, legumes, and whole grains, while some experts often combine IF with keto or low-carb or keto diet types. Assume that you will cope with lower stamina, cravings, and bloating before the body changes for the first several weeks.

Chapter 3:
Types of Intermittent Fasting

Several specific types of intermittent fasting exist. The most prominent ones include:

- The 16:8 method
- The warrior diet
- Time-restricted fasting
- Eat stop eat
- Spontaneous meal skipping
- The 5:2 diet
- Alternate-day fasting (ADF)

All intermittent fasting methods are beneficial and effective, but it depends on the individual to find out which works better.

3.1 16/8 Intermittent Fasting Method

One of the most favored forms of fasting for losing weight is the 16/8 intermittent fasting plan. Often it's called time-restricted fasting, though some variants are subtly different. A person fasts for 16 hours in the 16:8 model and restricts the eating to an 8-hour window of time. As a portion of the 16-hour window, several individuals miss breakfast. So, for instance, you could eat during the 12 pm to 8 pm range.

Some people, though, choose to miss supper instead. You could restrict the eating window to 9 am & 5 pm per day with this. To eat calories, a person can pick every 8-hour time and miss dinner or breakfast.

You might still eat the main meal a day for this fasting pattern. One can choose the timing of meals, like breakfast at 10:00 am, lunch will be at 2:00 pm, and dinner at 5:30 pm. By 6:00 pm, a person can finish eating their dinner so that all of the food consumption is done inside 10 am to 6 pm window, which is eight hours.

The fasting limits the consumption of calorie-containing drinks and food to a limited window of 8 hours a day. For the rest of the 16 hours of each day, it involves refraining from food. Whereas other diet plans can set rigid rules and regulations, the 16/8 process is more flexible and based on the time-restricted feeding (TRF) method.

This fasting model may help one lose weight and lower the blood pressure by limiting the number of hours that one can eat throughout the day. A review study found that the 16/8 technique helped decrease body fat and maintained muscle mass in several participants when coupled with physical exercise. A much more recent study showed that the 16/8 method did not hinder muscle gains in women performing aerobic exercise.

While the 16/8 technique can easily fit into every lifestyle, it may be difficult for some individuals to avoid eating 16 hours straight. Additionally, the potential benefits associated with 16/8 intermittent fasting can be negated by eating junk food or too many snacks during the 8-hour window. To maximize this intermittent fasting's health benefits, make sure to eat a healthy, balanced diet containing fresh vegetables, fruits, whole grains, good lean protein, and healthy fats.

3.2 The 5:2-Method of Intermittent Fasting

The 5:2 diet usually entails consuming normal amounts of calories to five days each week while reducing your calorie consumption for only 2 days of the week to 500-600 calories. Also known as the Fast Diet, this diet was popularized by British journalists. The 5:2 diet is a simple and direct intermittent fasting plan. You normally eat 5 days a week and don't limit your calories but also do not eat fried or unhealthy snacks. Then, you drop the calorie consumption to one-quarter of your standard requirements for the remaining two days of the same week. This means reducing the calorie intake to just 500 calories each day, 2 days per week, for someone who regularly consumes 2,000 calories each day.

According to research, for people with type 2 diabetes, the 5:2 diet is as efficient as daily calorie reduction for weight loss and blood sugar control. Another study showed that the

5:2 diet for both weight reduction and the treatment of metabolic disorders such as cardiac failure and diabetes was almost as successful as constant calorie restriction.

As the person gets to select the days they are fasting, the 5:2 diet promises versatility, and there are no guidelines on whether or what to consume on full-calorie days. Having said that, it should be remembered that eating "usually" on full-calorie days does not grant you a free pass to consume anything you want.

It's not convenient to restrict oneself to only 500 calories a day, even though it's just 2 days a week. And, you can feel sick or faint from eating very little calories. The 5:2 diet might be efficient, but it's not for everybody. In order to see if the 5:2 diet could be appropriate for you, speak to the doctor. There are days for low calorie, and you can eat around 25% of the calorie requirements, typically about 500 to 750 calories per day, and are sometimes referred to as "modified fasts."

It is recommended that women consume 500 calories on fasting days, and men consume 600. You can consume 2 regular meals of 250 calories per woman for two fasting days and 300 calories per man. No trials are evaluating the 5:2 diet itself, as opponents rightly point out, but there are loads of studies about the advantages of intermittent fasting.

- Low Carb Group 5:2 Intermittent Fasting has slightly larger decreases in insulin resistance and insulin relative to the low-calorie regular group. This category contained the most persons who had lost nearly 5% of their body weight.

- Low Carb Group with Fat and Protein Intermittent Fasting 5:2: lowered insulin and insulin resistance almost the same as the low-calorie regular group. This category has the lowest amount of weight reduction that came from fat. It makes sense as protein will try to stop fat burning(ketosis)

Furthermore, cholesterol levels, blood pressure, and inflammation were decreased for both classes. All intermittent fasting groups lost more body fat than the normal calorie restriction community. The investigators concluded that the IF 5:2 diet of fewer than 40 grams of carbohydrate a day produced the better outcomes of the three diets for body fat reduction and insulin sensitivity improvement.

3.3 Alternate-Day Intermittent Fasting

As the title suggests, every other day, alternate-day intermittent fasting is when one fast- or severely limits their caloric intake. For alternate-day fasting, a person fasts every other day. The alternative fasting method every other day is much less popular. Furthermore, trying it is perhaps the most difficult form of intermittent fasting. This fasting routine may not be feasible. As per the review study, it may lead to intense hunger on the fasting days. This other analysis revealed that most people who could do intermittent fasting were the respondents who tried to do alternative day fasting in an effort to lose weight. It also did not generate greater weight loss or maintenance of weight. Usually, this intermittent fasting is not strongly recommended. For the whole day, it is difficult not to eat. The person should worry about their blood sugar, levels of insulin, and energy. Your ability to think can also be disturbed. You are going to be extremely hungry.

A professor of nutrition popularized this strategy. This fast consisting of 25 % of one's calorie needs almost 500 calories. On non-fasting days to be typical eating days, people could fast every other day. This is a common approach to weight loss. In reality, alternative day fasting has been seen to help obese people who want to lose excessive weight. By two weeks, the adverse effects (like extreme hunger) diminished, and by four weeks, the participants continued to become more comfortable with the diet. The drawback of that during the experiment's eight weeks, respondents said they were never really felt their stomachs were full, which can make it difficult to adhere to this fasting method.

This intermittent fasting has several different versions. During intermittent fasting days, a few of them allow almost 500 calories. Some versions of this technique were used in many studies showing positive effects of intermittent fasting. A complete fast may seem far more extreme every other day, so it is not suggested for beginners. You can go to bed quite hungry several times a week with this method, that is not pleasant at all and, in the long term, probably unsustainable.

3.4 24-Hour fast/ One Meal a Day

Between meals, the trick is to fast for 24 hours. Eat at 7 pm on the first day, for example, and fast until 7 pm the following day. Conversely, a person can choose to eat earlier, either lunch or breakfast, and fast until the next day for 24 hours. The concept is that every day you eat a meal but allowing your body to fast for a longer period of time. This sort of fasting is usually performed once or twice a week, but it can be more frequently adopted. This type of fasting is not for everyone.

The OMAD intermittent fasting (one meal a day) is when one limits their eating window to only one hour per day, and for the remaining 23 hours, fasting happens. This is the ultimate type of intermittent fasting, and for many individuals, it can be an effective strategy for extreme weight loss.

Some of the risk factors of cardiovascular disease can be eased by this type of intermittent fasting but under strict medical supervision. During that window, one has to be able to last 23 hours without meals and resist the temptation to eat, as extreme hunger is a common complication of this sort of fasting.

3.5 Eat-Stop-Eat

Eat Stop Eat is an unorthodox approach to intermittent fasting popularized by an "Eat Stop Eat" journalist. This intermittent fasting plan includes classifying one or two non-consecutive days each week for a 24-hour cycle. During which one abstains from eating or fasting. one can eat freely during the remaining days of the week, but eating a well-rounded diet and avoiding overconsumption is suggested.

The reason behind a 24-hour fast every week is that eating fewer calories will ultimately lead to weight loss. Fasting for 24 hours can result in a metabolic shift that causes one's body to utilize stored fat rather than glucose as an energy source. But it requires a huge amount of self-discipline to avoid food for 24 hours on end and may lead to bingeing and excessive consumption later on. It may also result in eating disordered patterns.

In order to identify this pattern's potential health benefits and weight loss properties, much research is required regarding the Eat Stop Eat diet. Before attempting Eat Avoid Eat, speak with the doctor, and see if that could be an appropriate weight reduction solution for you. This strategy varies from other plans in that it emphasizes flexibility.

3.6 The Warrior diet

This intermittent fasting plan is called the warrior diet based on ancient warriors' eating patterns. The Warrior Diet, which was created in 2001, is a bit more dramatic than the 16:8 techniques but less rigid than Eat Stop Eats' method. It comprises eating almost nothing or very little during the day for 20 hours, then eating as much food as desired at night in a 4-hour eating window.

During the 20-hour fast period, the Warrior Diet promotes people to consume small quantities of hard-boiled eggs, dairy products, vegetables, and raw fruits and fluids with no calories. After the 20-hour fast, in a 4-hour eating window, individuals can eat anything they want, but it must be unprocessed. Organic foods and healthy are suggested. Although there is no research, especially on the Warrior Diet, studies show that time-restricted eating cycles can lead to weight loss.

There could be many other health advantages of time-restricted feeding periods. Studies indicate that feeding cycles that are time-restricted can inhibit diabetes, limit the development of tumors, postpone aging, and improve lifespan. More research on the Warrior Diet is needed to grasp its weight-loss advantages fully.

It can be challenging to adopt the Warrior Diet since it reduces significant calorie intake to only 4 hours a day. Excessive consumption of calories at night is a widespread problem. The Warrior Diet can often result in disordered eating habits. Speak to the doctor if you feel up to the warrior diet's task to see if it's correct for you. During the day, it means consuming tiny quantities of fresh fruits and vegetables and eating one big meal at night. Within a four-hour eating window, you fast throughout the day and dine at night. One of the first common diets to incorporate a form of intermittent fasting was the Warrior Diet.

This lifestyle's food preference is fairly close to that of the paleo diet, mainly unprocessed foods, whole foods. The Warrior Diet supports only tiny quantities of veggies and fruits to thrive throughout the day, then consume a big meal at night.

3.7 Spontaneous Meal Skipping

To enjoy any of its advantages, you don't need to adopt a formal intermittent fasting schedule. Another choice is to miss meals from time - to - time, such as cooking and eat and not consuming when you are too busy or don't feel hungry. It's a misconception that every few hours, people ought to consume calories before they enter hunger mode or lose their muscles. Your body is well prepared to cope with lengthy stretches of hunger, let alone the loss of one to two meals from time to time.

Therefore, one day you just don't feel hungry, miss breakfast, and only have a good lunch or dinner. Or, if you're going anywhere and you can't seem to find something you want to consume, do it easily and momentarily. It's simply a random sporadic quick to miss one or two meals anytime you are tempted to do so. Only make sure during the other meals to consume nutritious foods.

3.8 Choose-Your-Day Fasting

This is more of an adventure of your-own choice. Every other day or once or twice each week, you could do time-restricted fasting as you fast for 16 hours, and to eat for eight hours it means that Saturday could be a normal eating day, and by 8 p.m. one would stop eating; then at noon on Sunday, the eating will be resumed. It's like skipping breakfast several days a week.

3.9 Time-Restricted Fasting

You pick a feeding window every day with this form of Intermittent fasting, which will ideally leave a 14 to 16-hour fasting window. It is recommended for women over 50 to fast for no more than 14 hours each day due to hormonal issues. Fasting encourages autophagy, as discussed before, the simple and healthy cellular housekeeping process in which the body clears degenerated protein, cell debris, and other things that hinder the way of mitochondrial health, which begins when the body's glycogen is depleted, experts say. Doing it could help maximize the metabolism of fat cells and help optimize the function of insulin.

For this to work, a person may set their eating window from 9 a.m. To 5 p.m. This can work particularly well for somebody with a family who is still eating an early dinner. Far too much of the time spent fasting is still time spent asleep. Depending on that, when a person sets their eating window, you won't miss any meals. But this depends on how consistent one can be. If your schedule is very flexible, or you want the freedom to go out now and then for breakfast, or you want late dinners, it may not be for you to have daily fasting cycles.

3.10 Choosing Your Intermittent Fasting Plan

You may use a standard method that limits daily eating to a span of six to eight hours per day. For example, one may decide to try fasting for 16/8, eat for eight hours, and fast for 16 hours. Many experts are supporters of the daily regimen: that in the long run, most individuals find it convenient to adhere to this easy pattern.

Another approach is 5:2 strategies, which includes eating five days a week on a regular basis. One may restrict themselves to a daily 500 to 600 calorie meal for the rest of the two days.

Longer stretches without food are not inherently healthier for someone new to intermittent fasting, like 24, 36, 48, and 72-hour fasting periods, and can be risky. Going too long without eating could promote the body to start storing more fat in reaction to hunger and malnourishment.

Research suggests that intermittent fasting will take two to four weeks until the body becomes used to it. As you're becoming accustomed to the new schedule, you may feel hungry or grumpy. But, it says, study participants who make it past the time of transition prefer to adhere to the program, and they find that they feel healthier.

In deciding which intermittent fasting method is the best for you, your tolerance of hunger pangs can direct you. Although intermittent fasting for most active adults is usually safe, it is not intended for everybody.

Chapter 4:
Tips & Tricks on Getting Started with Intermittent Fasting for Women Over 50

Here are some tips and advice to get you started with Intermittent Fasting.

Stay hydrated. Drink plenty of beverages that are free of calories, such as water, herbal teas, during the day—avoiding a fascination with food. You must plan your fasting day around activities you enjoy, so you will not be thinking about food or obsessing over what you will eat next.

Resting & Relaxation. On fasting days, do not do strenuous exercises, while light physical activities such as yoga, walking around the house can be helpful.

Make each calorie count. Now that you have chosen a plan for intermittent fasting, it is necessary to eat every calorie as nutrient-rich as possible. Select foods that are rich in fiber, good lean protein, and healthy fats. Nuts, Corn, lentils, poultry, pork, fish, and avocado are some examples.

Consuming high-volume products. You must eat nutrient-packed high volume foods, but for snacking, also look for low-calorie foods such as melons, grapes, vegetables with high water content, fruits or popcorn

Improve the flavor without the calories. Generously season your meals with flavor-packed garlic, vegetables, sauces, or spices and fresh herbs. These spices are low-calorie but rich in flavor and will help in feeling the hunger less. Select foods that are nutrient-dense during fasting time.

Consuming diets that are rich in fiber, vitamins, minerals, and other nutrients tend to maintain blood sugar levels stable and avoid nutritional deficiencies. A healthy diet can also lead to weight reduction and good wellbeing. If you want to the 16:8 intermittent fasting, here are the tips that people find useful:

- Drinking herbal cinnamon tea throughout the fasting time because it can reduce the appetite

- Consuming water periodically during the day

- Watching minimal television to decrease sensitivity to food pictures that may stimulate a feeling of hunger

- Working out only before or during the feeding window, since exercise will contribute to hunger

- Try to eat thoughtful nutrition-packed food after breaking fast. Try meditation to encourage hunger pangs to pass throughout the fasting time.

Speak to your doctor if you're thinking about attempting intermittent fasting, particularly if you already have health problems such as heart conditions and diabetes. Expert advises trying to take it easy with the diet. The time window for feeding is shortened steadily over many months.

Also, as the specialist has advised, continue the medication routine. It doesn't interrupt the fast to take drugs, and take the medication with calorie-free beverages like black coffee and water.

- What if you require food with medicines?

You may try to modify the fast in that case. It has been shown that overweight individuals can always do a lot of good even by taking medication with small portions of food. Simply work out a prescription with your practitioner that would support your wellbeing without losing the benefits.

You would like to ease into whether you are planning to attempt a fat fast or do intense intermittent fasting. If you are already consuming an unhealthy diet packed with quick snacks, fatty foods, and refined carbohydrates, you don't want to rush into these extreme fasts. One will find themselves in the bathroom for much of the day if you try to rush into fasting. Instead, by first performing a 16:8 fast on its own and keeping off the junk food, build your way up to doing these intense ways of intermittent fasting. Some literature speaks of doing a fat fast over a few days up to several weeks at a time.

- Your subconscious is the greatest barrier.

It's really easy to follow this plan. You simply should not eat until you wake up. Then you have lunch and dinner, and then you go on your day.

- Weight loss is simple.

If you consume less frequently, you will prefer to eat less in general. As a consequence, most people that pursue intermittent fasting wind up losing weight. You might be preparing large meals, but in reality, consuming them regularly is tough. Keep monitoring what healthy foods make you feel better during fasting and keep cycling them. Intermittent fasting helps, but before a person incorporates carb cycling and calorie cycling, some people did not lose weight. By consuming a lot on the days you exercise and eat less on the days you do not exercise, you cycle calories.

- Prepare to get a lot of water to drink.

For you, the safest lifestyle is the one that fits for you.

4.1 Pay Attention to These Things When Starting Intermittent Fasting Over 50

One might find themselves grappling with hunger pangs as of a fasting novice. Don't worry; once the body gets used to intermittent fasting, these are going to vanish. Ensure that one drinks enough water, particularly throughout the fasting window, during the day. Water can help keep headaches at ease, which will encourage you to stay feeling full. Tea, black coffee, and low sodium bone broth are other drinks you can drink. Remember not to add milk or sugar to coffee and tea, or you fast won't do you any good.

Until you have achieved your fast, do not be pressured to overeat. Plan in advance: Load the plate with fresh, nutrient-packed foods full of high-quality lean proteins, fiber, and good fats instead of bingeing on anything in view. After the fast is over, these healthy meals will hold you sated and less inclined to overeat.

Here are some frequently thought out questions for people over 50.

During the fast, can one drink liquids? Yes. It is good to have water, tea, black coffee, and other non-caloric drinks. Do not add the cream to coffee. There could be tiny quantities of milk or cream that are okay. They must be non-fattening. During a fast, coffee may be especially helpful, as it can curb hunger.

Is missing breakfast unhealthy? No. The concern is that there are unsafe lifestyles for most traditional breakfast skippers. If you make sure that for the remainder of the day, you consume nutritious food, so fasting is healthy.

When fasting, should one take supplements? Yes. Bear in mind, though, that certain supplements can function best when taken with meals, such as fat-soluble vitamins, so look out for that.

Can an individual exercise while fasting? Yes, easy workouts are okay. But remember not to overexert yourself. For women over 50, simple yoga, brisk walking around the house, cleaning also count as work out. Yeah, easy workouts are okay.

Would fasting trigger muscle loss? All forms of weight reduction can induce muscle loss, so lifting weights and maintaining your protein consumption is crucial. One research found that intermittent fasting induces less loss of muscle than a daily restriction of calories.

Can The Metabolism Slow down during Fasting? No. Studies indicate that short-term fasting improves metabolism. Lengthier fasts of three or more days, therefore, can suppress and disrupt metabolism.

Chapter5(A):
Foods to Eat & Avoid in Intermittent Fasting

Here are some nutrition-packed foods one should consume to help with hunger pangs and keep your belly full for a longer time.

5.1 Food List of Lean Proteins

Consuming lean protein can leave one feeling fuller for longer than eating other diets. It also helps in retaining or construct muscle. Here are some forms of lean, balanced protein:

- Plain Greek yogurt.
- Beans, peas & lentils.
- Tofu & tempeh
- Fish & shellfish.
  - Chicken breast.

5.2 Food List of Fruits

It is essential to consume fully nutritious foods during intermittent fasting, just like in any other eating routine. Minerals, vegetables, and fruits are packed with Vitamins, nutrients from plants, and fiber. These nutrients, vitamins, and minerals can help lower the amount of cholesterol, regulate blood sugar, hypertension, and maintain the intestines' function. There are low-calorie vegetables and fruits available.

The Nutritional Recommendations suggests that most people should consume around two cups of fresh fruit on a regular basis for a 2,000 calorie diet. Through intermittent fasting, here are some good fruits to eat

- Apricots.

- Watermelon.
- Blueberries.
- Plums.
- Cherries.
- Peaches.
- Apples.
- Pears.
- Oranges.
- Blackberries.

5.3 Food List of Vegetables

A major portion of an intermittent fasting plan is to consume vegetables. Research suggests that the risk of heart failure, cancer, type 2 diabetes, cognitive impairment, and more can be minimized by a diet rich in leafy greens. The Nutritional Recommendations suggest that most people should consume two and a half cups of vegetables on a regular basis for a 2,000 calorie diet.

As part of a balanced intermittent eating routine, here are some vegetables that will be nice to consume:

- Kale.
- Collard greens.
- Spinach.
- Cabbage.
- Arugula.
- Chard.

5.4 Carbs for Intermittent Fasting

- Avocado
- Sweet potatoes
- Oats
- Apples
- Brown rice
- Mangoes
- Bananas
- Quinoa
- Almonds
- Berries
- Chia seeds
- Pears
- Carrots
- Beetroots
- Broccoli
- Kidney beans
- Chickpeas
- Brussels sprouts

5.5 Fats for Intermittent Fasting

- Avocados
- Dark chocolate
- Nuts
- Whole eggs
- Fatty fish
- Cheese

- Full-fat yogurt
- Extra virgin olive oil
- Chia seeds

5.6 Beverages for Hydration in Intermittent Fasting

- Sparkling water
- Watermelon
- Strawberries
- Oranges
- Water
- Cantaloupe
- Peaches
- Lettuce
- Celery
- Black coffee or tea
- Tomatoes
- Cucumber
- Skim milk
- Plain yogurt

There are some foods you must include in your intermittent fasting schedule:

5.7 Water

Essentially, water is not food, but it's essential one to get through IF. Basically, for any significant organ in the body, water is vital to wellbeing. As part of the fast, you will be reckless to stop drinking water. The organs are pretty significant. Depending on gender, height, activity level, weight, and environment, the amount of water each person can drink differs. But a reasonable indicator is your urine color. For all times, you like it to be pale yellow.

Dehydration indicates dark yellow urine, which may induce headaches, exhaustion, and lightheadedness. Couple it with minimal food, and you've got a catastrophe formula, or rather dark pee, for the very least. Add a splash of lemon juice, some few mint leaves, or any cucumber slices to the water if the prospect of pure water does not excite you. Promoting hydration is among the most critical ways of sustaining a balanced eating routine when fasting intermittently.

When you go for 12-16 hours without food, the sugar contained in the liver, also known as glycogen, is the main source of energy for the body. When this energy is burned, A huge amount of electrolytes and fluid dissolve. During the intermittent fasting regimen, consuming at least 8 cups of water a day can reduce dehydration and encourage improved cognition, blood flow, and joint muscle and support.

5.8 Coffee

What about a nice cup of hot coffee? Do not worry; Coffee is allowed. Since coffee is a calorie-free product in its natural form, it may also be drunk beyond a specified feeding window. But if you add creamers, syrups, or any flavorings, it cannot be drunk at the duration of the fast. Keep that in mind and enjoy coffee

5.9 Less-Processed Grains

When it comes to weight control, carbohydrates are an important aspect of life. They are most certainly not the enemy. Since a significant part of the day would be spent fasting, it is necessary to carefully think of ways to get enough calories while not feeling too full. A balanced diet minimizes refined foods, but products such as whole-grain bagels, bread, and crackers may have time and location, as these foods are digested more easily for fast and convenient fuel. If a person plans to work out or frequently exercise while fasting intermittently, this would be a fantastic energy source on the go in particular.

5.10 Raspberries

In the Dietary Recommendations, fiber was designated a deficient ingredient, and a recent report in Nutrients reported that less than ten % of populations eat sufficient amounts of whole fruits. Raspberries are a tasty, high-fiber fruit with eight grams of fiber each cup to keep you well-nourished during the fasting window.

5.11 Lentils

With 32% of the daily total fiber requirements fulfilled in just half a cup, this healthy superstar packs a high fiber impact. In addition, lentils provide a great iron source, another important nutrition, particularly for active women experiencing intermittent fasting.

5.12 Potatoes

White potatoes are metabolized with minimum effort in the body, close to bread. They are a great post-workout snack to recharge hungry limbs if combined with a protein source. Another advantage that makes these an essential staple for the Intermittent Fasting diet is that potatoes have resistant starch that is prepared to fuel healthy bacteria in the gut.

5.13 Hummus

Hummus is another great plant-based protein, one of the tastiest and creamiest dips known to man, and is a perfect way to improve the nutritious value of classics such as burgers, replace with mayonnaise. If you're bold enough to make hummus at home, don't overlook that tahini and garlic are the keys to a good recipe.

5.14 Wild- Salmon

Salmon, which is rich in omega-3 fatty acids, brain-boosting DHA & EPA, is one of the nutrients widely eaten in the whole worldwide.

5.15 Unprocessed Soybeans

Iso-flavones are one of the active compounds in soybeans, have been proven to prevent cell damage by UVB-and facilitate anti-aging, as well as being impeccable in taste. So, you must include soybeans at your dinner parties.

5.16 Multivitamins

The fact that the person actually has much less time to eat and therefore consumes less is one of the suggested mechanisms behind why IF contributes to weight loss. While the concept of energy in vs. energy out is valid, the possibility of vitamin deficiency while in a dietary deficiency is not always addressed. And a healthy diet of lots of fruits and vegetables, while a multivitamin is not mandatory, life can get hectic, and vitamin supplementation can fill the nutrition gaps.

5.17 Fresh Smoothies

Try jumping to a double dose of vitamins by making organic smoothies filled with fresh vegetables and fruits if a daily supplement doesn't suit you. Smoothies are a perfect way to ingest diverse foods, each filled with various essential nutrients, especially. Buy frozen fruits to save money and for ultimate delicious recipes.

5.18 Fortified Milk with Vitamin D

The average calcium consumption is 1,000 mg a day for an adult, exactly what you can receive from consuming three cups of milk a day. The opportunities to drink this much may be scarce with a shortened feeding window, so it is necessary to choose high-calcium foods. Vitamin D fortified milk increases calcium absorption by the body. It helps maintain bones healthy. one should add milk to cereal or smoothies or even just consume it with foods to improve the regular calcium intake. Non-dairy options rich in calcium contain tofu and soy goods, as well as leafy greens, including kale.

5.19 Blueberries

Don't be misled by their tiny size. Blueberries assure that tiny packets come with decent goods. Studies have demonstrated that anti-oxidative pathways are the product of youthfulness and longevity. Blueberries are a perfect source of antioxidants. One of the main sources of antioxidants is wild blueberries. Antioxidants help to get rid of free radicals in the body and stop widespread cellular destruction.

5.20 Papaya

One will usually begin to feel the consequences of hunger during the final hours of the fast, particularly when you first start intermittent fasting. In exchange, this hunger can lead one to overeat in substantial quantities, leaving the person feeling sluggish and bloated minutes later.

Papaya has a special enzyme called papain that helps to break protein down by working on them. It will help ease digestion by using pieces of this tropical fruit is a protein-packed meal, keeping some bloating more manageable.

5.21 Nuts

Leave space for a mixed variety on the cheese plate since nuts in all kinds are believed to remove body fat and lengthen your lifespan. Prospective research reported in the Journal of Nutrition also connected the decreased incidence of coronary disease, type 2 diabetes, and total mortality to nut intake.

5.22 Ghee

You've learned, of course, that a drizzle of olive oil has substantial health benefits, but there are lots of other oil alternatives out there that one can still use. If you are not comfortable to heat the oil cook to beyond the flames' point, think of using ghee as a substitute for preference the next time cooking up a stir-fry.

5.23 Homemade Dressing Salad

When one talks about sauces & salad dressings, you can keep it homemade just as your grandma kept her food wholesome and easy. Unwanted ingredients and added sugar are removed as we choose to produce our basic dressings.

Chapter 5(B):
Superfoods to Eat for Women Over 50
In Intermittent Fasting

5.24 Avocado

Eating the highest-calorie food when attempting to lose weight can seem strange. Although, because of its high content of unsaturated fat, avocados can make you feel full throughout the day, even the longest times of fasting. Even when a person doesn't feel full, evidence shows unsaturated fats help hold your body feel full. The body sends signals that it has adequate calories and will not move into hunger mode in an emergency. Unsaturated fats hold these signals running for longer, even though you get a little hungry during a fasting time. Another research also showed that it could keep you satisfied for hours. so you must add these green mushy fruit to your diet during intermittent fasting

5.25 Fish & Seafood

There is a cause that the Nutritional Recommendations suggest that two or three servings of 4 ounces of fish be consumed each week. It includes sufficient quantities of vitamin D, besides being high in good fats and protein. If you eat during fasting with small windows, don't you want to eat nutrition-packed food. There are many ways to enjoy fish that one can never run out of ideas.

5.26 Cruciferous Vegetables

Broccoli, cauliflower, and Brussels sprouts are full of the most important nutrition fiber. It's essential to consume fiber-rich foods that keep the body regular and make the gut function smoothly, especially when you eat after intervals. Fiber may also help one to feel full, which might be a positive thing if you can't eat for 16 hours. Cruciferous vegetables may also minimize cancer risk.

5.27 Potatoes

As mentioned before, potatoes are one of the heartiest food to eat, that will keep you full, as the main course or snack or in lunch during intermittent fasting. Not all foods that are white and starchy bad for you. But French fries and potato chips do not count as healthy options.

5.28 Legumes & Beans

In the IF lifestyle, the favorite addition to chili maybe your best mate. Food, including carbohydrates, offers energy for physical activity. It is not asked of you to carb-load to insane amounts, but tossing some low-calorie carbohydrates like legumes and beans into the diet plan will certainly not cause any harm. During the fasting hours, this will hold you active, and without calorie limits, foods such as black beans, chickpeas, peas, and lentils are shown to lower body weight.

5.29 Probiotics

Do you know what good bacteria want the most in the gut? Diversity & consistency. That implies that when they are hungry, they aren't content. And you can feel certain annoying side effects, including constipation, while the stomach isn't content. Add probiotic-rich products such as kefir, sauerkraut, and Kombucha to the diet to combat this discomfort.

5.30 Eggs

6.24 grams of protein is provided by one big egg and cooked up in minutes. And it is important to get as much protein as needed to sustain fullness and build muscle, particularly when one eats less. Women who had an egg breakfast rather than a bagel are far less hungry and ate less during the day, a 2010 study showed. In other terms, why not hard-boil those eggs while you're hunting for anything to do during the fasting period? And, when the time is perfect, you should enjoy them.

5.31 Whole Grains

It appears like going on a diet and consuming carbohydrates fit in two separate buckets. To realize that this is not necessarily the case, you'll be super happy. Whole grains supply plenty of nutrition and fiber, but eating less goes a long way to keep yourself full. So do not hold back from whole-grain like bulgar, farro, bulgur, spelt, Kamut, amaranth, millet, freekeh, or sorghum, from your comfort place.

Other nutrition-packed superfoods are nuts, blueberries as they are already discussed prior.

5.32 Foods to Avoid During Intermittent Fasting

To do intermittent fasting correctly, many things are not healthy to eat. You can keep away from foods that contain huge amounts of salt, sugar, and fat that are calorie-dense. These foods won't fill you up fast, and they might also leave you hungry. They have little or no nutrients, as well.

Avoid these ingredients to sustain a safe intermittent feeding regimen:

- Processed foods
- Snack chips.
- Refined grains
- Trans-fat
- Alcoholic beverages
- Sugar-sweetened beverages
- Microwave popcorn.
- Candy bars
- Processed meat

In addition, you must avoid foods that are rich in added sugar. Sugar is devoid of any nutrients and contributes to sweet, hollow calories in the form of refined foods and beverages, which is what you should avoid while you're intermittently fasting. Because the sugar metabolizes super-fast, it will make you even hungrier.

You should avoid these sugar-packed foods if you are trying to do intermittent fasting:

- Frosted Cakes.
- Cookies
- Sugar added Fruit juice.
- Candies
- Sugary cereals and granola
- Barbecue sauce and ketchup.

Foods such as nuts, lean proteins, seeds, fresh vegetables, and fruits should be your main focus during intermittent fasting as they help in weight loss and help keep your stomach full.

To prevent any nutritional deficiencies, healthy eating is the key to successful intermittent fasting.

Chapter 6:
Mistakes to Avoid During Intermittent Fasting

When it comes to intermittent fasting for beginners, it is necessary to avoid these misconceptions and mistakes no matter your age.

6.1 Rushing into Intermittent Fasting

You are more likely to get hungry all the time and discouraged if you are regularly eating every 3 to 4 hours and then unexpectedly shrink your mealtime to only 8 hours. According to some experts, any individuals will stop intermittent fasting if they start by fasting for many hours without a transition time from a prior eating style. It can take between 10 days to 2 weeks for someone to quit feeling hungry when they fast. One of the greatest errors you can create is to start dramatically.

You can set yourself up for failure if you dive into IF without easing into it. It may be not easy to move from consuming 3 regular sized meals or 6 tiny meals per day to eating only within 4 hours.

Instead, ease slowly into fasting. If you are going for the 16/8 technique, progressively increase the period between meals so you can operate inside 12 hours comfortably. Then, add multiple hours a day before you get to the 8-hour window.

There are levels of intermittent fasting. The primary factor most diets don't harvest benefits is their drastic deviation from our normal, usual eating habits. Sometimes, it can seem not easy to sustain. You think about it if someone is new to IF, then they're used to eating every 2 hours, you are going to very uncomfortable during long hours of fasting. It is normal to have a transition time, but it should feel better.

A remarkably strong communicator is the body itself. If it feels like trouble, it will let you know. And it is a common fact that you are going to feel like crap to starve yourself out of literally nowhere for 23 hours.

If you are stubborn about the principle of fasting, begin with the 12:12 approach of a beginner: fast for 12 hours a day and feed in the next 12-hour window.

That's pretty similar to what a person is used to doing nowadays, and who knows that it could be the only practical way to pursue it. You should level up to 16:8 once it seems comfortable, where you consume over an 8-hour window and fast during the remainder of the day. The best thing about IF is its simplicity, so choose a schedule that encourages you to adhere to a time frame without feeling bad. The number of hours one go between meals is slowly extended until they hit a 12-hour feeding time. Then switch to an eating window of 10 hours and decrease by tiny amounts before meeting your target.

6.2 Expecting Intermittent Fasting to Change Your Life

Another error people seem to make is that they make their lives more about fasting than living. Because someone is fasting, they don't need to turn down the dinner request from their mates or a birthday celebration. That is not going to make it less satisfying and can still maintain such a lifestyle. Instead, on days where you have commitments with people, move your day backward or forward by a couple of hours so you can always enjoy socializing.

Note, there is versatility in intermittent fasting.

6.3 Choosing The Wrong Fasting Plan for Yourself

If you are trying something that would make your lifestyle difficult, it's not going to be the best option. Don't sign yourself up for disappointment fasting only for few days, then going back to your previous unhealthy ways won't be good for you. It's about adjusting the lifestyle you can maintain over a long time. Don't try to start the fast at 6 p.m. if someone is a night person. If someone is a regular gym-goer, then pick a fasting schedule that will suit your style.

Anyone else does not know your lifestyle. The specialist is you. And you have to make changes that if you want to stick to the fasting pattern. If one is ready to pursue

Intermittent Fasting and look for whole grains and healthy food such as fish, chicken and fruits, vegetables, and nutritious sides such as tofu, legumes, and quinoa for weight loss, then fasting will benefit you. The issue is, if you haven't picked the right IF strategy, it will not give you success. Like if you are a committed gym-goer six days each week, the perfect schedule might not be to fast entirely on two of those days.

6.4 Not Drinking Enough and Drinking the Wrong Stuff

One intermittent fasting error to avoid is consuming the wrong drinks and not drinking sufficiently while fasting. Even if it is calorie-free, you don't want to consume something that's overly sweetened. Since it also has a detrimental impact on insulin levels and will stimulate your appetite and make yourself want to snack.

When fasting, aim to stick to water, pure tea, or black coffee. If one does not drink sufficiently, it may also cause dehydration, contributing to headaches, muscle cramps, and exacerbating hunger pangs.

6.5 Overeating When Fasting Ends

Overeating after completing the fast is another famous error. When a fast end, it may be simple to overeat simply because one may feel ravenous, or people justify themselves because they made up for missed calories, which is why they overeat.

But if you're fasting for weight reduction especially, this may turn out badly and even trigger some issues, including stomach aches. Prepare your meals beforehand; when your fast finishes, cook a nutritious recipe that is available for you and ensure that you consume whole foods wherever possible, including healthy carbohydrates such as seafood, vegetables, lean protein, and whole grains.

To avoid this, all you have to do is schedule your day, including the fasting and eating period ahead, ensuring that you eat healthy and keto-friendly foods after breaking the fast.

6.6 Eating Too Much in The Fasting Window

Most of the time, people want to pursue Intermittent Fasting is because it involves eating fewer calories; it means they also will have less time to eat. In the duration of the fasting window, though, certain individuals will consume their normal amount of calories. This will imply you are not going to lose weight. Do not consume the normal intake of calories in the window. Rather, when one breaks the fast, expect to consume about 1200 to 1500 calories. If it is 4, 6, 8 hours, how much meals one can consume would depend on the duration of the fasting window.

If you need to overeat and are in a condition of starvation. Reconsider the strategy you want to adopt, or relax off the IF for a day to regroup and then get back on board

6.7 Forcing It On Your Self

Forcing the body to fast is yet another error. It is necessary to note that it is not for everybody to start intermittent fasting. It's all right to re-assess if this is the best strategy for you. Yes, some say that our bodies will cope quite frequently with hunger, but that doesn't imply that it's the best thing for everyone to do right now.

Not all bodies are developed for intermittent fasting. Ask yourself this easy question if intermittent fasting seems like a relentless challenge and emotional drain: Is the compromised standard of life worth it?

6.8 Not Paying Attention to The Nutrient Quality of the Foods

When following intermittent fasting, people often rely on fast foods when they simply concentrate on what to eat more than what they should consume. Instead of keeping a well-balanced diet, if you continue with refined foods, you should not anticipate intermittent fasting to achieve your fitness goals. By adopting nutritious foods steadily, aim to adjust your lifestyle along with your meal routine progressively.

6.9 Restricting The Food Intake Too Much

Not eating sufficient and going too far with fasting. You've got to note that fasting isn't for starving. Our bodies need fuel to move around, work properly, think straight, and converse naturally, and that fuel comes from food. It takes a toll on daily life to limit your food consumption so much, and that's not the main concern of what fasting is all about.

The what is overlooked in favor of the when. IF is a time-centered diet, and most schedules do not include any clear guidelines during the feeding window for the kinds of food to consume. Although this is not an accessible invitation for French fries, beer, and milkshakes, to thrive. Fasting isn't magic. In addition to certain minor physiological effects, the main influence on weight reduction is that you minimize the hours of feeding and the number of calories you eat.

If you've already had a pre-workout snack, it can sound alien to exercise when fasting. But when there are no calories, the body has loads of resources left in the body fat to use. As for every diet or workout schedule, consulting with the doctor first is a smart practice, but with intermittent fasting, exercising may be healthy.

Keep up with your normal fitness regimen or do something like cycling that is low-impact. You should consume a protein-rich meal after that. Always make sure to consult with your doctor first as over 50 you should not do strenuous exercises while fasting

Sadly, by selecting the wrong types of foods, you cannot easily reverse the influence. During the feeding hours, change your mindset from a "treating yourself" attitude to one that centers around consuming the most nutrient-packed, nourishing meals you can find. To better fill yourself up and carry you during the fasting process, we suggest making sure any meal or snack contains a mix of fiber, protein, and good fats.

- Cook all the meals at home and try not to eat takeout's or in restaurants

- Pay attention to nutrition labels and make sure to not consume forbidden ingredients like modified palm oil, corn syrup, high fructose

- Try to consume low sodium and beware of added sugar

- Do not eat processed foods and home cook whole foods

- Add fiber, good fats, and fiber to your plate, and lean proteins

Chapter 7:
Exercises to do with Intermittent Fasting in Women Over 50

Forms of Exercise: Two forms of exercise, aerobic and anaerobic, are essential. Exercise for a prolonged time, such as racing, biking, and swimming, is physical exercise, or 'cardio' Anaerobic training, such as weight lifting or sprinting, involves full intensity for a limited time.

The type of exercise an individual performs is likely to depend on the type of intermittent fasting they practice. For instance, an individual doing nightly fasts or 16:8 will do either anaerobic exercise or aerobic exercise during their eating while not over-exerting themselves.

If anyone does alternate days and wishes to work out on their day of fasting, they should usually adhere to physical exercise less severe. Two main things to look out for if you want to try an exercise with intermittent fasting.

- **Timing of the workout:** While an individual can work out in a fasting state, it may be easier to exercise after meals.

- **Sort of food:** It is necessary to know what to consume while exercising throughout times of consumption.

Nutrition of Pre-workout consists of consuming a meal 2-3 hours before doing exercise rather than just before exercising. It should be high in complex carbs, such as protein and cereal from whole grains.

A Post-Workout Meal should consist of fresh vegetables, good quality proteins, and fats to facilitate healing.

For some people over 50, fasting and exercising daily might be dangerous, including:

- People who had disordered eating

- People with low blood pressure
- People with a heart condition
- People with diabetes

If an individual has just worked out: the meal they consume should be 50 to 60 % of the calories in this situation and have a mixture of macronutrients.

If an individual is working out later: the meal they consume should be 30 to 50 % of the calories in the meal, made up of a combination of macronutrients.

When an individual has existing health problems but needs to try Intermittent fasting and workout, it is better to speak to the doctor.

7.1 Light movement exercise during intermittent fasting include:

- Rather than laying or sitting still, light movement is good

- Get up and making a cup of coffee and tea,

- Moving around the building

- Strolling at a steady speed

- Dusting and washing

- Vacuuming activities

- Make your bed

- Walking and standing then walking

- Yoga

7.2 Examples of moderately intense activities:

- Water aerobics

- Riding a bicycle

- Walking briskly

- Dancing like exercise

- Hiking on a hill

- Playing doubles tennis

- Push a lawnmower

These are some excises that women over 50 can also try with intermittent fasting

- Aerobic exercise includes running, jogging, walking, cycling, and dance activity are good things to do. The aerobic activity works with the body's broad muscles, aiding the cardiovascular system, and losing weight. Work up to having 20 minutes or more, a session, 3 to 4 days each week. Be sure one can pass the "talk test," which involves exercising at a speed that lets you continue on a conversation.

- Strength exercises. Lifting hand weights strengthens stamina and balance, improves bone strength, decreases the likelihood of lower back injuries, and makes you fit. Begin with a hand weight that one can easily handle for eight repetitions. Add more reps progressively before you can total 12.

- Stretching: Stretching movements aim to preserve joint stability and range of motion. They often reduce the likelihood of muscle soreness and injuries. Pilates and yoga is a good way of stretching exercise, strengthening the core body, and enhancing flexibility.

Chapter 8:
Overcoming Down Moments in Intermittent Fasting

When it comes to one's ultimate health and desire to achieve the targets, controlling appetite, and keeping healthy food is important. Intermittent fasting will help you accomplish this, but although certain individuals can fast with very little problem for long stretches, some people can find it a bit more challenging, particularly when they first start.

There is a set of ideas to help you out that one can use to get the best results and make the ride a little smoother.

8.1 Start the Fast After Dinner

One of the best advice one can offer is when you do regular, or weekly fasting is to begin the fast after dinner. Using this ensures you're going to be sleeping for a good portion of the fasting time. Especially when using a daily fasting method like 16:8

8.2 Eat More Satisfying Meals

The type of food one consume affects their willingness to both the urge to complete the fast and what you crave to eat after the fast. Too much salty and sugary foods with making you hungrier rather than consume meals that are homey satisfying and will help you lose weight

- Morning eggs or oats porridge

- A healthy lunch of chicken breast, baked sweet potato, and veggies.

- After the workout, drink a protein milkshake.

- Then you end the day in the evening with an equally impressive dinner.

8.3 Control Your Appetite

Without question, while fasting, hunger pangs can set in from start to end. The trick as this occurs is to curb your appetite, and with Zero-calorie beverages that help provide satiety and hold hunger at bay before it's time to break the fast, the perfect way to do this is. Examples of food to consume are

- Sparkling water

- Water

- Black tea

- Black coffee

- Green tea

- Herbal teas and other zero-calorie unsweetened drinks

8.4 Stay Busy

Boredom is the main threat. It is the invisible assassin who, bit by bit, creeps in to ruin the progress, breaking you down steadily and dragging you downwards. For a second, think about it. How often boredom has caused you to consume more than you can, intend to, or even know that you are. Hence try to plan your day.

8.5 Stick to A Routine

Start and break your fast each day at regular times. Consuming a diet weekly where you finish similar items per day. Meal prepping in advance. Making a plan allows things easier to adhere to the IF schedule, so you eliminate the uncertainty and second-guessing the process until you learn what works for you and commit to it every day. Follow-through is what one has to do.

8.6 Give Yourself Time to Adjust

When one first starts intermittent fasting, odds are you're going to mess up a couple of times; this is both OK and natural. It's just normal to have hunger pangs. This doesn't mean that you have to give up or that it's not going to be effective for you. Alternatively, it's a chance to learn, to ask whether or how you messed up, and take action to deter it from occurring again.

8.7 Enjoy Yourself

Let yourself enjoy the process. No one starts at the pro level, so you should go out with your friends and attend those birthday parties as well.

Chapter 9:

Intermittent Fasting Appetizers, Sides & Snacks Recipes

9.1 Berry Crisp

(Ready in about: 45 minutes | Serving 6)

Ingredients

Fruits

- 1 teaspoon of cinnamon
- ¼ cup of milk, nonfat
- 1 bag of (16 ounces) cherries or bag of blueberries
- Half teaspoon of nutmeg
- 1 box of (7/8 ounce) jello vanilla-flavor, sugar-free, pudding mix, cooked

Crisp

- One cup of plain fat-free yogurt
- 1 and a half cups of old fashioned oats
- Almond extract: 1 teaspoon
- Half cup of Splenda sugar substitute

Instructions

- Take an 8by8 baking pan.
- In a pan, add all fruits and mix well.
- In another bowl, add all ingredients of crisp. Mix well.
- Add this mix over the berry mix so that it will be the top crust.
- Bake for 40 to 45 minutes, at 350 F, or until the top gets lightly browned and crunchy.

Nutrition per serving: **one of 6 servings:** Calories: 121.6| Total Fat 1.5 g| Cholesterol 1 mg| Calories from Fat 13 g| Total Carbohydrate 22 g| Sugars 7.6 g| Protein 5.2 g| Sodium 34.6 mg|

9.2 Broccoli Dal Curry

(Ready in about: One hour and 30 minutes | Serving 4)

Ingredients

- Unsalted butter: 4 tablespoons or 4 tablespoons of ghee
- Chili powder: 1 teaspoon
- Cumin: 2 teaspoons
- Ground coriander: 1 teaspoon
- Two medium-sized onions, finely chopped
- Turmeric: 2 teaspoons
- 1 and a half teaspoons of freshly ground black pepper
- Red lentil: 1 cup, cleaned and rinsed
- Fresh juice from one lemon
- Low sodium chicken broth: 3 cups
- All-purpose flour: 1 tablespoon
- Broccoli: 2 medium-sized, chopped
- Half cup of dried coconut (it is optional)
- Cashews: 1 cup, roughly chopped (it is optional)
- Half teaspoon of salt

Instructions

- In a pan, add butter and onions, sauté until tender and browned
- Add turmeric, chili powder, black pepper, coriander, and cumin. Cook for one minute.
- Add broth, lentils and lemon juice, coconut. Stir well

- Let it boil, turn the heat down to low and let it simmer for 45 to 55 minutes. Add water if the lentil is too thick.
- In a steamer over boiling water, place broccoli, steam for 7 minutes.
- Wash steamed broccoli with cold water and set it aside.
- Take out 1/3 cup of mixture from lentils. Mix with flour to make a paste.
- Pour back in the pot, add salt, nuts, and broccoli.
- Let it Simmer for five minutes.
- Serve with rice and enjoy.

Nutrition per serving: one of 4 serving: Calories: 445| Total Fat 15.4 g| Cholesterol 30.5 mg| Sodium 362.4 mg | Dietary Fiber 15.1 g| Sugars 8.5 g| Protein 25.7 g| Total Carbohydrate 59 g|

9.3 Sweet Potato & Black Bean Burrito

(Ready in about: One hour and 15 minutes | Serving 8-12)

Ingredients

- Half teaspoon of salt
- 2 teaspoons of extra virgin olive oil or 2 teaspoons of low sodium broth
- 3 and a half cups of onions, diced
- 5 cups of sweet potatoes, peeled, cut into cubes
- 4 cloves of minced garlic
- Green chili pepper, freshly minced: 1 tablespoon
- Fresh lemon juice: 2 tablespoons
- Ground coriander: 4 teaspoons
- Ground cumin: 4 teaspoons
- Four and a half cups of cooked black beans
- Fresh salsa
- 2/3 cup of lightly packed leaves of cilantro

- 12 flour tortillas of (10 inch each)

Instructions

- Let the oven preheat to 350 F
- In a pot, add enough water to cover sweet potatoes and salt. Add sweet potatoes.
- Cover the pot let it simmer for ten minutes.
- Drain the potatoes and set it aside.
- In a pan, add olive oil, over medium flame, sauté garlic, chili and onions.
- Cover it and cook for 7 minutes on low heat until onions become tender.
- Add coriander, cumin cook, for 2-3 minutes, stirring often.
- Turn off the heat and set it aside.
- Add cilantro, cooked sweet potatoes, lemon juice, black beans, and salt in a food processor.
- Pulse on high until pureed.
- Take the mixture out in a bowl. And mix in the sautéed onions.
- Grease a baking dish with light oil.
- Add 2/3-3/4 cup of black bean mixture in every tortilla, roll tightly, and put in a baking dish, seam side down.
- Cover with aluminum foil and cover for half an hour.
- Add fresh salsa on top and serve.

Nutrition per serving: Calories: 575.2| Calories from Fat 92 g| Cholesterol 0 mg| Sodium 416.4 mg | Sugars 8.7 g | Protein 19.8 g| Total Carbohydrate 102 g| Dietary Fiber 15.9 g|

9.4 Almond Lentil Stew

(Ready in about: 50 minutes | Serving 3-4)

Ingredients

- 1 diced carrot
- 1 diced stalk of celery
- Extra virgin olive oil: 2 tbsp.+ one teaspoon for the almonds
- 1 finely chopped turnip
- 2 cloves of minced garlic
- 1 finely chopped onion
- One cup of baby button mushrooms, cut into halves
- One and ¼ cup of green lentils
- 4 cups of lows sodium vegetable stock
- Ground cinnamon: 1 tbsp.
- One bay leaf
- Ten cherry tomatoes, cut into quarters
- Four sprigs of thyme
- Handful of almonds
- One sprig of rosemary

Instructions

- In a pan, add 2 tsp. of olive oil, heat the oil, and sauté onion, carrot, turnip, and celery. Cook for five minutes, until tender.
- Add mushroom and garlic—cook, for more than five minutes.
- Add lentils, cook for one minute and add herbs, stock. Let it boil, then turn the heat down to low, let it simmer for 45 minutes.
- After 40 minutes, in another pan, add one tsp of oil and almonds with cinnamon—Cook for two minutes.
- Add cherry tomatoes and cook for 2-3 minutes.

- In a bowl, add lentil stew, sprinkle with toasted tomatoes, and almonds.

Nutrition per serving: one cup: Calories: 256 | Total Fat 12 g| Total Carbohydrate 19.8 g| Dietary Fiber 3 g| Sugars 4.5 g| Protein 13.4 g| Sodium 213 mg|

9.5 Toasted Crumpets &Warm Spiced Berries with Yogurt & Honey

(Ready in about: 15 minutes | Serving 2)

Ingredients

- ¾ cup of ripe strawberries, cleaned and cut into slices
- Four crumpets
- Half cup of fat-free Greek yogurt
- ¼ cup of blueberries
- Ground mixed spice: 3 pinches
- ¼ cup of raspberries
- Runny honey: 2 teaspoons, for serving

Instructions

- Grill or toast the crumpets until crispy and browned.
- In a bowl, add yogurt and whisk until it looks shiny and glossy.
- In a pan, over medium flame, add all fruits. Add pinches of ground spice mix, and cook for one minute, until fruits start to become tender. This step is necessary for the sweetness of fruits without adding any sugar.
- Add hot toasted crumpets to 2 plates. Add fruits on top. Pour yogurt and drizzle with honey.

Nutrition per serving: Calories: 230.7| Total Fat 11.4 g| Total Carbohydrate 15.4 g| Dietary Fiber 2.4 g| Sugars 12.7 g| Protein 3.4 g| Sodium 241 mg|

9.6 Coconut Vegan Banana Kefir Muffins

(Ready in about: 45 minutes | Serving 12)

Ingredients

- Dried shredded coconut, unsweetened: 1 cup
- All-purpose flour: 2 cups
- Grainy sugar: 1 cup or sugar alternative
- Low sodium baking powder: 1 teaspoon
- 1 and a half cups of kefir probiotic, dairy-free, coconut milk, fermented
- Low sodium baking soda: 2 teaspoons
- 1/8 teaspoon of salt
- 1/4 cup of liquid coconut oil, cold-pressed
- 2 ripe bananas, mashed
- Vanilla extract: 1 teaspoon

Instructions

- Let the oven preheat to 350 F. Spray muffin tin with cooking spray and set it aside.
- In a bowl, add coconut, baking powder, flour, sugar, salt, and baking soda. Mix well.
- In a big bowl, add vanilla, bananas, coconut oil, and kefir mix to combine.
- Add in the flour mix, mix until well combined.
- Add to a prepared muffin tin and bake for half an hour until inserted toothpick comes out clean.
- Let the muffin tin tray cool for 12-15 minutes.

Nutrition per serving: one muffin: Calories: 300.7| Total Fat 15.4 g| Total Carbohydrate 39.7 g| Dietary Fiber 2.2 g| Sugars 19.7 g| Protein 3.4 g| Sodium 344 mg| Cholesterol 0 mg|

9.7 French Vanilla Almond Granola

(Ready in about: 2 hours and 10 minutes | Serving 12)

Ingredients

- 3 and a half cups of old fashioned oats (not the quick oats)
- Half cup of water
- ¼ cup of organic canola oil
- Half cup of natural cane sugar
- ¼ teaspoon of salt
- Vanilla extract: 1 tablespoon
- Half cup of almonds, cut into slices

Instructions

- Let the oven heat to 200 F. place large parchment paper on a rimmed baking sheet.
- In a bowl, add almonds, oats mix well.
- In a pan, add salt, water, and sugar on medium flame mix well. Cook until sugar dissolves.
- Turn off the heat, add in vanilla, and canola oil. Add in almond, oats mixture, and mix until combined.
- Pour mixture on a prepared baking sheet and bake until dry or for 2 hours, do not mix.
- Take out from the oven. Let it cool, then break into large pieces.
- Keep safe in an air-tight container.

Nutrition per serving: one big piece: 187.1 Calories | Total Fat 8 g| Sodium 50.4 mg| Total Carbohydrate 25.3 g| Saturated Fat 0.7 g| Sugars 8.8 g| Protein 3.9 g|

9.8 Spicy Chocolate Keto Fat Bombs

(Ready in about: 8 minutes | Serving 24)

Ingredients

- Smooth peanut butter: 2/3 cup
- Half cup of dark cocoa
- Coconut oil: 2/3 cup
- 4 packets of stevia each (6 g), (or to taste)
- Ground cinnamon: 1 tablespoon
- Cayenne pepper: 1/4 teaspoon
- Kosher salt: 1/4 teaspoon
- Half cup of coconut flakes, toasted

Instructions

- In a double boiler bowl over simmer hot water, add cocoa powder, coconut oil, and peanut butter. Whisk until smooth.
- Add salt, stevia, and cinnamon mix to combine.
- Pour mixture in a mini silicone muffin tray, or place liners in a muffin tin.
- Sprinkle cayenne and coconut.
- Let it freeze for half an hour.
- Serve and enjoy.

Nutrition per serving: one fat bomb: 110 Calories | Total Fat 10.3 g| Sodium 62.2 mg| Saturated Fat 6.5 g| Sugars 1.3 g| Cholesterol 0 mg| Protein 2.2 g| Total Carbohydrate 3.6 g|

9.9 Avocado Quesadillas

(Ready in about: 30 minutes | Serving 2)

Ingredients

- Two ripe tomatoes, remove seeds cut into 1/4 inch of pieces
- Half teaspoon of vegetable oil
- One ripe avocado, peel it, remove the pit, diced into 1/4 inch pieces
- Fresh lemon juice: 2 teaspoons
- Tabasco sauce: ¼ teaspoon
- Red onion, chopped: 1 tablespoon
- Salt and pepper, to taste
- Sour cream: ¼ cup
- 24" of tortillas (flour)
- 1 and ⅓ cups of Monterey Jack cheese, shredded
- Freshly chopped coriander: 3 tablespoons

Instructions

- In a bowl, add onion, Tabasco, tomatoes, lemon juice, and avocado. Mix well.
- Season with salt and pepper, to taste.
- In another bowl, add sour cream, black pepper, coriander, salt to taste, and mix well.
- Place tortillas on a baking sheet and drizzle with little oil
- Broil the tortillas 2-4 inches from heat until lightly golden.
- Add shredded cheese on tortillas, and broil again till cheese melts.
- Add the avocado mixture to 2 tortillas and place one tortilla on top. Put cheese side down.
- Take out the quesadillas to a cutting board and cut it into four pieces.
- Put the sour cream mix on top and serve.

Nutrition per serving: one tortilla: 794.9 Calories | Total Fat 51.1 g| Cholesterol 82 mg| Sodium 678.8 mg| Saturated Fat 21.6 g| Total Carbohydrate 58.7 g| Sugars 7.2 g| Protein 29.2 g|

9.10 Shredded Brussels Sprouts with Bacon & Onions

(Ready in about: 30 minutes | Serving 6)

Ingredients

- 4 cups of Brussels sprout, cleaned and trimmed, cut into halves, thinly sliced
- 2 slices of bacon
- One small-sized, yellow onion, cut into thin slices
- 3⁄4 cup of water
- Dijon mustard: 1 teaspoon
- 1⁄4 tsp. of salt

Instructions

- In a large pan, add bacon over medium flame, cook until crispy for 5-7 minutes, drain and then crumble, absorb excess grease with a paper towel.
- Add salt to taste and onion, add drippings to the pan, and cook for three minutes until soft, browned, and tender.
- Add mustard, water mix well, then add Brussels sprouts, cook for 4-6 minutes.
- Add in vinegar and sprinkle with the crumbled bacon.
- Serve and enjoy.

Nutrition per serving: one of six serving: 45.2 Calories | Total Fat 1.6 g| Cholesterol 1.8 mg| sodium 145.9 mg| Saturated Fat 0.5 g| Total Carbohydrate 6.5 g| Protein 2.4 g| Dietary Fiber 2.2 g|

9.11 Roasted Broccoli with Lemon-Garlic & Toasted Pine Nuts

(Ready in about: 22 minutes | Serving 4)

Ingredients

- 4 cups of broccoli floret
- Unsalted butter: 2 tablespoons
- Extra virgin olive oil: 2 tablespoons
- Salt & freshly ground black pepper
- Toasted pine nuts: 2 tablespoons
- Half teaspoon of freshly grated lemon zest
- Fresh lemon juice: 1 -2 tablespoon
- Minced garlic: 1 teaspoon

Instructions

- Let the oven preheat to 500 F
- In a mixing bowl, add oil, broccoli, salt, and pepper. Toss well.
- Add tossed broccoli and roast for 12 minutes on a baking sheet, flipping once halfway through until tender.
- In a pan, add melted butter over medium flame.
- Add lemon zest, garlic, and sauté for one minute. Let it cool slightly.
- Add in the fresh lemon juice.
- In a bowl, add roasted broccoli and pour over lemony butter.
- Toss well.
- Sprinkle pine nuts on top.

Nutrition per serving: one of 4 servings: Calories: 172.7| | Total Fat 15.8 g| Cholesterol 15.3 mg| Sodium 31.8 mg| Dietary Fiber 0.2 g| Protein 4.1 g| Total Carbohydrate 7 g| Sugars 0.3 g|

9.12 Vegan Lentil Burgers

(Ready in about: One hour and 10 minutes | Serving 8-10)

Ingredients

- Extra virgin olive oil: 1 tablespoon
- 2 and a half cups of water
- Dry lentils: 1 cup, rinse well
- Half teaspoon of salt
- Half of a medium chopped onion
- Fresh ground black pepper: 1 teaspoon
- One carrot, finely diced
- Rolled oats: ¾ cup, finely ground
- Breadcrumbs: ¾ cup
- Light soy sauce: 1 tablespoon

Instructions

- In salted boiling water, add lentils, and boil for 45 minutes, or until they are soft and all the water is absorbed.
- In a pan, add olive oil over medium flame, sauté carrots, onions until soft, for five minutes.
- In a bowl, mix the cooked lentils, carrots, and onion with soy sauce, breadcrumbs, black pepper, and oats.
- Form patties while the mixture is still warm enough to handle. Make 8 to 10 patties.
- Bake them for 15 minutes at 200 C or shallow fried for 1 to 2 minutes on each side until browned and cooked through.

Nutrition per serving: Serving Size: one patty: 176.4 Calories | Total Fat 3 g| Sodium 354.9 mg |Total Carbohydrate 28.5 g| Sugars 1.9 g| protein 9 g| Dietary Fiber 9 g|

9.13 Vegan Pancakes

(Ready in about: 45 minutes | Serving 4-6)

Ingredients

- Coconut oil: two tbsp.

- Baking powder: 2 tsp.

- Salt: 1/4 tsp

- White whole-wheat flour: One & a half cup.

- Unsweetened almond milk: 1 and 1/2 cup

- Unsweetened applesauce: 1/4 cup

- Sugar: 1 tbsp.

- Vanilla extract: 1 tsp

Instructions

- In a wide bowl, mix in the salt, flour, and baking powder. In a medium dish, whisk together the vanilla, applesauce, milk, oil, and sugar.

- Create a well in the middle of the dry ingredients, incorporate the wet ingredients, and whisk until done. don't overmix. — it will make the pancakes hard.

- Let the batter stay there for fifteen minutes, without stirring.

- Cover the large skillet with oil spray over medium flame.

- Measure pancakes utilizing around 1/4 cup batter per pancake without stirring the batter and drop in the pan.

- Cook for 2 to 4 minutes until the sides are dried and bubbles on the top. Flip and cook on the other side for 2 to 4 minutes, until golden brown. Repeat the process and serve.

Nutrition Per Serving: 174 calories| fat 4.1g| carbohydrates 6.8g | protein 5.8g | total fat 31.6g | carbohydrates 8 g |fiber 12 g |

9.14 Quinoa & Chia Oatmeal Mix

(Ready in about: 10 minutes | Serving 12)

Ingredients

- Quinoa one cup
- Rolled oats: 2 cups
- Dried fruit: 1 cup
- Barley flakes: 1 cup
- Chia seeds: half tablespoon
- Salt: 3/4 cup
- Ground cinnamon: one teaspoon

Instructions

- Combine nuts, barley flakes, dried fruit, Quinoa, salt, and cinnamon in an airtight jar to create the hot cereal dry mix

- To produce one serving of hot cereal: add 1/3 of a cup of Quinoa and dry mixture of Chia Oatmeal in a tiny saucepan with milk or water. Let it simmer. Reduce heat, cover, and boil, frequently stirring for fifteen minutes until thickened. Let wait for five minutes, covered up.

- If needed, stir in a sweetener, and finish it with dried fruits or nuts.

Nutrition Per Serving: Calories 194 |Fat: 10g|Carbohydrates: 22g|Fiber: 6g| total fat 12 g | carbohydrates 9.4g | protein 18.6g|

9.15 Steel Cut Oats with Kefir & Berries

(Ready in about: 30 minutes | Serving 4)

Ingredients

- Steel-cut oats: 1 cup
- Water: 3 cups
- Unsweetened kefir
- Salt: a pinch

For toppings

- Frozen fruits or berries
- Maple syrup or artificial sweetener
- Sliced nuts

Instructions

- In a small saucepan, add the oats and put over medium to high heat. Let them toast, swirl, or shake the skillet for three minutes.
- Then add the water to get it to a boil. Reduce heat, and let it steam for around 25 minutes, or until the oats are soft enough. (The oats thicken as they cool — if you want them to be like a little more porridge, add more water or milk)
- Serve with the fruit, nuts/seeds (or a pinch of granola), a drizzling of kefir, and sweetener you like

Nutrition Per serving: Calories 240| Fat: 18g| Net Carbs: 7g| Protein: 17g| total fat 10 g | carbohydrates 5.6 g |fiber 2.5g |

9.16 Chai-Spiced Buckwheat & Chia Seed Porridge

(Ready in about: 20 minutes | Serving 6-8)

Ingredients

- Milk: 2 cups
- Buckwheat 1 cup
- Chia seeds: 2 tablespoons
- Oats: ½ cup
- Water: 2 cups
- One grated apple
- One grated pear
- One teaspoon of ginger and cinnamon(powder)
- Nut butter: 2 tablespoons
- Honey: 2 tablespoons
- Half teaspoon of nutmeg and cardamom(powder)
- Vanilla extract: 1 teaspoon

Berry Compote(Mixed)

- Water: 1 tablespoon
- Mixed frozen berries: 500 g
- Caster sugar: ⅓ cup
- Corn flour: 2 teaspoons
- Juice of one orange and its zest

Instructions

- In a bowl, place the buckwheat and oats, and fill with cold water.
- Place the chia seed in a separate cup and add 1 cup of milk.
- Leave the two bowls for an overnight soak.
- In a fine sieve, drain the buckwheat and oats, then wash well under cold water.

- Put the chia seeds in a medium saucepan with the remaining 1 cup milk, buckwheat, oats, sugar, grated pear and apple, and all the spices, butter, honey, and vanilla.
- Cook for around 30 minutes over low heat, sometimes stirring until smooth and fluffy, adding more water or milk to hold it at a soft consistency.
- Serve with toppings of your likings in bowls.

Nutrition Per serving: Calories 240| Fat: 12g| Net Carbs: 7g| Protein: 20g| total fat 11.6g | carbohydrates 9.4g |fiber 2.7g | Phosphorus 143 mg

9.17 Gluten-Free Buckwheat Pancakes

(Ready in about: 25 minutes | Serving 8)

Ingredients

- Sugar: 1 tablespoon
- Baking powder: one teaspoon
- Salt: ¼ teaspoon
- Buckwheat flour: 1 cup
- Buttermilk: 1 ¼ cups
- One egg
- Vanilla extract: ½ teaspoon
- Baking soda: one teaspoon
- Oil spray

Roasted Strawberries

- Sugar: 1 teaspoon
- Strawberries halved: 1 pint
- Honey to drizzle

Instructions

- Strawberries to roast: let the oven preheat to 350 F. place parchment-papered on a baking sheet. Tossing berries lightly in a small bowl with the maple syrup. Put the strawberries over the baking sheet in one layer. Let it roast for half an hour.

- Making of the pancakes: combine all the flours, baking powder, sugar, salt, and baking soda in a bowl. Measure the buttermilk. Mix the vanilla extract with egg.

- Combine the dry ingredients with the wet ingredients, mix well.

- Let your skillet heat with 1 ½ teaspoon butter over medium flame. If the buckwheat is beginning to separate from the batter, give the batter a light swirl with a spoon.

- Put the batter in the warm pan, using a ¼-cup measure. Cook for three minutes till you see small bubbles form on the pancake's surface and flip over. Cook for two more minutes.

- Put the pancakes on a baking tray and put them to keep warm in a preheated 200 F oven.

- Remove from oven and serve.

Nutrition Per serving: Calories 140| Fat: 12g| Net Carbs: 3g|Protein: 17g| total fat 31.6g | carbohydrates 9.4g |fiber 2.5g | Phosphorus 113 mg

Chapter 10:
Intermittent Fasting Poultry & Meat Recipes

10.1 Herb-Roasted Chicken Breasts

(Ready in about: 40 minutes | Serving 4)

Ingredients

- One onion

- 4 cups of chicken breasts (boneless and skinless)

- 1–2 cloves of garlic

- Ground black pepper: 1 teaspoon

- Olive oil: ¼ cup

- Garlic & Herb Seasoning: 2 tablespoons (no salt added)

Instructions

- In a bowl, chop garlic, onion, add herb seasoning, olive oil, and pepper.

- Add chicken to this mix, cover with plastic wrap, then chill in the fridge for four hours.

- Let the oven preheat to 350 F

- Place marinated chicken on foil on a baking tray

- Add the marinade over chicken and bake for 20 minutes

For browning

- Broil for five minutes.

Nutrition Per Serving: Calories 270 | total Fat 17 g| Cholesterol 83 mg| Sodium 53 mg| Carbohydrates 3 g| Protein 26 g| Phosphorus 252 mg| Dietary Fiber 0.6 g|

10.2 Zesty Chicken

(Ready in about: 30-40 minutes | Serving 2)

Ingredients

- Olive oil: 2 tablespoons

- Balsamic vinegar: 2 tablespoons

- Green onion: 1/4 cup

- Paprika: 1/4 teaspoon

- 8 ounces of chicken breast (skinless and boneless)

- Black pepper: 1/4 teaspoon

- Fresh oregano: 1 teaspoon

- Half teaspoon of garlic powder

Instructions

- In a mug, whisk olive oil and balsamic vinegar. Add chopped green onion, herbs, and seasoning, mix well. Cut chicken into two pieces.

- In a zip lock bag, add chicken and pour marinade over. Let it chill in the fridge for half an hour to 24 hours.

- Grease the pan, cook chicken until chicken's internal temperature reaches 170 F

Nutrition per serving: Calories 280| Protein 27 g| Carbohydrates 4 g| Fat 16 g| Cholesterol 73 mg| Sodium 68 mg| Calcium 26 mg| Fiber 0.3 g

10.3 Chicken Quinoa Anti-Inflammatory

(Ready in about: 45 minutes | Serving 4)

Ingredients

- Olive oil divided: 4 tbsp.

- Boneless, skinless chicken breasts: one pound

- Finely chopped red onion: ¼ cup

- Roasted red peppers: 2 cups

- One minced garlic clove

- Paprika: 1 tsp.

- Crushed red pepper: ¼ tsp(optional)

- Cooked quinoa: two cups

- Ground cumin: half tsp.

- Olives, chopped: ¼ cup

- Diced cucumber: one cup

- Almonds: ¼ cup

- Crumbled feta cheese: ¼ cup

- Salt: ¼ teaspoon

- Ground pepper: ¼ teaspoon

- Fresh parsley: 2 tbsp.

Instructions

- In the upper third of the oven, put a rack; let the broiler preheat. Place foil on a rimmed baking dish.

- Put salt and pepper on the chicken, and put on the prepared baking sheet. Broil it for 14 to 18 min, rotating once, till a thermometer instant-read added in the thickest section registers 165 degrees F. Move the chicken and slice on a cutting board.

- Meanwhile, put two spoons of oil, cumin, peppers, almonds, crushed red pepper in a food processor. Pulse it until creamy

- In a medium dish, mix olives, quinoa, two spoons of oil, and red onion. mix it well

- Divide the quinoa mixture into four bowls and finish with similar quantities of red pepper sauce, cucumber, and tomato to eat. Sprinkle with parsley and feta.

- Enjoy.

Nutrition Per Serving: 219 calories| total fat 26.9g |carbohydrates 31.2g |protein 34.1g | Potassium 187 mg| Phosphorus 132 mg

10.4 Skillet Lemon Chicken & Potatoes with Kale

(Ready in about: 40 minutes | Serving 4)

Ingredients

- Chopped tarragon: one tbsp.

- Boneless, skinless chicken thighs: one pound(trimmed)

- Ground pepper: half tsp. Divided

- Olive oil: 3 tbsp.

- Salt: half tsp. divided

- Light chicken broth: half cup

- Baby kale: 6 cups

- One lemon; sliced

- Four cloves of garlic(minced)

- Baby Yukon Gold potatoes: one pound; halved lengthwise(leached)

Instructions

- Let the oven pre-heat till 400 F.

- In a large skillet, heat one tbsp. of oil.

- Sprinkle with 1/4 teaspoon of salt and pepper on chicken. Cook, rotating once, before browning on both sides, a total of about 5 minutes. Move into a tray.

- Add 1/4 tsp. of salt and pepper to the pan with the remaining two teaspoons of oil, with potatoes.

- Cook potatoes, cut-side down, for around 3 minutes, until browned. Add lemon, broth, garlic, and tarragon. Bring the chicken back into the pan.

- Switch the frying pan to the oven.

- Roast, about 15 minutes, before the chicken is completely cooked and the potatoes are soft.

- Stir the kale into the mixture and roast for 3 to 4 minutes until it has wilted.

Nutrition per Serving: Calories 347 | total fat 19.3g |carbohydrates 25.6g | protein 24.7g | Potassium 171 mg| Phosphorus 151 mg

10.5 Grilled Chicken Salad with Mango & Avocado

(Ready in about: 25 minutes | Serving 4)

Ingredients

- One and a half cup of chicken breast, grilled and sliced

- Red onion, diced: 2 tablespoons

- Diced mango: 1 cup

- Baby lettuce, red butter: 6 cups

- Diced avocado: 1 cup

Vinaigrette

- White balsamic vinegar: 2 tablespoons

- Olive oil: 2 tablespoons

- Half tsp of turmeric

- Fresh ginger: ¾ tsp

Instructions

- In a bowl, add all ingredients of vinaigrette, whisk well and set it aside.
- In another bowl, add chicken, mango, onion, and mango. Toss together.
- In a serving platter, add baby greens on the bottom, add tossed salad on top, and drizzle with vinaigrette.
- Toss and serve right away.

Nutrition per serving: one bowl: 321 calories| sodium 154 mg |protein 28.4g | fat 7.1g | carbohydrates 31 g |cholesterol 28 mg

10.6 Chicken & Snap Peas Stir Fry

(Ready in about: 30 minutes | Serving 2-3)

Ingredients

- Skinless chicken breast: 1 and ¼ cups (sliced)

- Vegetable oil: 2 tbsp.

- Two minced garlic cloves

- Snap peas: 2 and ½ cups

- Black pepper and salt

- Cilantro: 3 tbsp. and for garnish

- One bunch of scallions (thinly sliced)

- Low sodium Soy sauce: 3 tbsp.

- One red bell pepper(sliced)

- Sriracha: 2 tsp.

- Sesame seeds:2 tbsp.

- Rice vinegar: 2 tbsp.

Instructions

- Heat the oil over medium flame in a large pan. Stir in the garlic and scallions, then sauté for around one minute until fragrant. Stir in the snap peas and bell pepper, then sauté for 2 to 3 minutes until soft.

- Add the chicken and cook for 4 to 5 minutes until golden and thoroughly cooked, and the vegetables are tender.

- Add the sesame seeds, soy sauce, rice vinegar, Sriracha, mix well to blend. Allow boiling the mixture for two minutes.

- Add the cilantro and garnish with coriander and sesame seeds. Serve hot

Nutrition Per serving: 228 calories|11g fat|11g carbs|20g protein| Potassium 210 mg| Phosphorus 105 mg

10.7 Chicken Caprese Sandwich

(Ready in about: 35 minutes | Serving 2-3)

Ingredients

- Extra virgin olive oil: 4 tablespoons, or more, divided

- Half lemon juiced

- ¼ cup of sliced fresh basil leaves

- Kosher salt and freshly ground black pepper

- One log of fresh mozzarella cheese of8 ounces, sliced into rounds (1/4 thickness)

- Skinless: 2 pieces of boneless chicken breasts

- Fresh parsley: 1 teaspoon(sliced)

- One loaf of ten ounces' sourdough bread, cut in half lengthwise

- Balsamic glaze or balsamic vinegar, to taste

Instructions

- In a big mixing bowl, add parsley, black pepper, two tablespoons of extra virgin olive oil, salt, lemon juice, mix it well. Pour this over chicken breasts and toss lightly to coat well, and let the chicken rest at room temperature.

- Put a grilling pan over medium heat. Add the chicken breast to the grilling pan, without the marinade, and add black pepper and salt. Flip the chicken after four minutes.

- Cook for three minutes more, till grill marks appear.

- Lower the flame, and cover the chicken and cook till the instant-read thermometer reads 185 degrees.

- Turn off the heat and slice the chicken, and set it aside.

- Pour one tablespoon of extra-virgin olive oil to each side of the bread and grill it until golden brown.

- Slice the bread into three slices for each half. Add 3-4 slices of chicken, few slices of mozzarella cheese to each slice. Pour balsamic vinegar, extra virgin olive oil on top. Add basil leaves on top.

- Season with more salt and black pepper.

- Serve hot

Nutrition per serving: calories 321 g| Fat 32.06g|Carbohydrates 46.88g|Protein 34.42g| Potassium 210 mg| Phosphorus 125 mg

10.8 Zucchini Noodles with Pesto & Chicken

(Ready in about: 20-25 minutes | Serving 4)

Ingredients

- Boneless, skinless: 4 cups of chicken breast, cut into bite-size pieces

- 1/4 cup extra-virgin olive oil and two tablespoons more

- Four pieces of trimmed medium-large zucchini

- ¼ of cup shredded Parmesan cheese

- Fresh basil (packed) leaves: 2 cups

- Lemon juice: 2 tablespoons

- One large clove of chopped garlic

- ¼ of cup toasted pine nuts

- Half teaspoon of freshly ground black pepper

- ¾ of teaspoon kosher salt, divided

Instructions

- Cut the zucchini in length into big, thin strands, utilizing a spiral vegetable slicer. Chops these long noodles so the strands would not be very long. Put the zucchini in a colander, and add 1/4 teaspoon of salt. Let it drain for almost half an hour, then press gently to extract any remaining moisture.

- In a food processor bowl, add Parmesan, basil, 1/4 teaspoon of salt, pine nuts, 1/4 cup of olive oil, black pepper, lemon juice, and garlic, and pulse on high until smooth

- Put a wide skillet over medium flame, add one tbsp. of oil. Add chicken in an even layer, then add 1/4 teaspoon of salt.

- Let it cook, often stirring, for about 5 minutes. Then transfer to a bowl and stir in three tablespoons of the pesto.

- To the pan, add the remaining one tablespoon of olive oil. Then add the dried zucchini noodles mix carefully for two-three minutes.

- Add these noodles to the bowl with the cooked chicken. Add the leftover pesto and toss lightly to coat.

Nutrition per serving: 430 calories| total fat 31.6g | carbohydrates 9.4g |fiber 2.5g |protein 28.6g| Potassium 187 mg| Phosphorus 143 mg

10.9 Keto Chili

(Ready in about: 60-65 minutes | Serving 7-8)

Ingredients

- Ground beef: 10.8 cups

- Celery: 2/3 cups, diced

- Red capsicum: 1/2 cup, diced

- Green capsicum: 1/2 cup diced

- Yellow onion: 1 1/2 cups, diced

- 1 cup chopped tomatoes

- Tomato juice: 1 1/2 cups

- Can crushed tomatoes in puree: 2 cups

- Worcestershire sauce: 1 and 1/2 teaspoons

- Chili powder: 3 tablespoons

- 2 teaspoons erythritol, granular

- 1 teaspoon Sea salt

- 1 teaspoon of garlic (powder)

- 1 teaspoon of cumin

- 1/2 teaspoon of oregano

- 1/2 teaspoon of black pepper

Instructions

- Brown the ground beef in a big bowl until it is cooked. Save about two spoonsful of Fat and drain the remainder of the Fat.
- Put the garlic, celery, black bell peppers, and tomatoes into the beef bowl. Cook for another five minutes, over medium-high heat.
- Add tomato juice, the diced tomatoes, the Worcestershire sauce, and all the seasonings. Cover and cook for 1 to 1 1/2 hours, sometimes stirring.

Notes (additional)

- Ten minutes before serving, uncover, and remove from heat. To top with shredded cheddar cheese and finely diced onions if desired.

Nutrition per serving: Calories 225 |Carbs 7 g |Protein 10 g |Fat 12g| carbohydrates 9.4g | Potassium 137 mg|

10.10 Lettuce Wraps

(Ready in about: 20 minutes | Serving 3-4)

Ingredients

For Lettuce Wraps

- Minced turkey: 3.6 cups
- Olive oil: 1 tablespoon

- 2 teaspoon of dried minced onion
- 1/4 teaspoon of sea salt
- 1/4 teaspoon of black pepper
- 3 green onions, thinly sliced
- ¼ cup chopped shiitake mushrooms
- 1/2 cup of diced jicama
- Living butter lettuce

Sauce's ingredients

- 3 tablespoon of soy sauce (less sodium)
- Two cloves garlic should be minced
- 1/2 teaspoon of ginger paste
- 1 teaspoon of sesame oil
- 1 teaspoon of rice vinegar
- One teaspoon of brown Swerve sweetener
- 1 teaspoon of almond butter, natural

Instructions

- Put all ingredients in a small bowl, whisk, and set aside.
- Heat olive oil in a skillet on the stove. Crumble and cook the minced turkey on medium heat.
- Season with chopped onion, sea salt, and black pepper.
- Then add green onion, jicama, and mushrooms.
- Add mushroom with meat until mushroom becomes soft—mix sauce with meat mixture.
- Serve.

Nutrition per serving: Calories 188 |Proteins 26g |Carbs12g |Fat 12g |Fiber 5g| carbohydrates 9.4g | Potassium 157 mg|

10.11 Grilled Chicken Breast

(Ready in about : 30 minutes| Serving 2)

Ingredients

- Chicken breasts: 4 pieces

For the Margination

- Olive oil: 3 teaspoon
- Cilantro chopped ¼ cup
- Garlic minced two cloves
- One lime juice
- Cumin: 1/2 teaspoon
- Sea salt: ½ teaspoon
- Paprika: ½ teaspoon
- Black pepper: ¼ teaspoon

Avocado Salsa

- Two small chopped tomatoes
- Red onion: ¼ cup chopped
- One jalapeno
- Cilantro: 1/4 cup finely chopped
- Diced avocado: two
- One lime, juiced
- Sea salt and black pepper

Instructions

- In a bowl, add all ingredients of marinade. Mix well and set it aside.

- With a meat mallet, pound the chicken breast, and add to the marinade. Coat the chicken well in the marinade. Keep in the fridge for half an hour or overnight if you have time.

- Preheat the grill pan over medium flame. Cook chicken for 5 to 6 minutes on each side or until cooked through and looks crispy on the outside.

- Serve right away with avocado and fresh salsa and enjoy.

For Salsa Avocado

- In a bowl, add all ingredients of salsa. Meanwhile, the chicken is cooking. With plastic wrap, cover it and keep in the fridge till serving time.

- It is one of the delicious and the easiest recipes to make.

Nutrition per serving: Calories 468 |Proteins 20g |Carbs 15g|Fat 10g |Fiber 2g| total fat 31.6g | carbohydrates 9.4g | Potassium 187 mg| sodium 91 mg

10.12 Cheesy Chicken Salad

(Ready in about: 35 minutes | Serving 1-2)

Ingredients

- Skinless, boneless chicken breast, cooked: 1 cup, cut into cubed

- 2 and a half tablespoons of mayonnaise, fat-free

- Finely chopped celery: ¼ cup

- Half cup of fresh baby spinach, coarsely chopped

- Sour cream, non-fat: 2 tablespoons

- Carrot: ¼ cup, shaved to ribbons

- Dijon mustard: 2 teaspoons

- Sharp cheddar cheese, reduced-fat: ¼ cup, shredded

- Dried parsley: 1/8 teaspoon

Instructions

- In a mixing bowl, add all ingredients. Mix all ingredients well with mayonnaise mixture.

- Keep in the fridge for half an hour, or overnight if you prefer.

- Serve and enjoy.

Nutrition per serving: 364.5 Calories | Total Carbohydrate 15.3 g| Total Fat 9.1 g| Cholesterol 131.8 mg| Dietary Fiber 2.8 g| Sugars 7.3 g| Protein 53.2 g| Sodium 767.4 mg|

10.13 Chicken Breasts with Avocado Tapenade

(Ready in about: 15 minutes | Serving 4)

Ingredients

- Fresh lemon juice: 5 tablespoons, divided

- Extra virgin olive oil: 3 tablespoons divided

- 2 cloves of garlic, roasted and then mashed

- 1 clove of finely chopped garlic

- Freshly grated lemon peel: 1 tablespoon

- 1/4 teaspoon of salt

- 4 skinless, boneless chicken breast cut in halves

- Fresh ground black pepper: half teaspoon

- 1 tomato, medium-sized, remove seeds, finely diced

- 1 ripe avocado, large-sized, finely diced

- Capers: 3 tablespoons, rinsed

- fresh basil leaves: 2 tablespoons, cut into fine slices

- ¼ cup of small-sized green pimento olive stuffed, cut into thin slices

Instructions

- In a zip lock bag, add 2 tbsp. of lemon juice, garlic, black pepper, 2 tbsp. of olive oil, ¼ tsp. of salt, lemon peel, and chicken. Mix well and keep in the fridge for half an hour.

- In a bowl, add roasted garlic, ¼ tsp of salt, half tsp of olive oil, 3 tbsp. of lemon juice, black pepper. Mix and add in basil, green sliced olives, avocado, tomato, capers. Set it aside.

- Take out the chicken from the bag, discard the marinade.

- Preheat the grill on medium flame and cook chicken for 4-5 minutes on each side or until cooked through.

- Serve grilled chicken with avocado salad.

Nutrition per Serving: one out of 4 servings: 277.1 Calories | Cholesterol 75.5 mg| Total Fat 16.4 g| Sodium 914.6 mg| Dietary Fiber 3.1 g| Protein 26.4 g| Total Carbohydrate 6.9 g|

10.14 Lemony Chicken Kale Orzo Soup

(Ready in about: 40 minutes| Serving 6

Ingredients

- Chicken broth: 4 cups

- Chicken breasts: one pound (1-inch pieces)

- Dried oregano: 1 tsp.

- Olive oil: 2 tbsp.

- Salt: 1 and ¼ tsp.

- Diced onions: 2 cups

- One bay leaf

- Orzo pasta: 2/3 cup

- Diced celery: 1 cup

- Chopped kale: 4 cups

- Two minced cloves of Garlic

- Diced carrots: 1 cup

- One lemon juice and zest

- Black pepper: ¾ tsp.

Instructions

- Heat one tbsp. of oil over medium flame in a big pot. Add the chicken, oregano (1/2 teaspoon), salt, pepper. Cook for five minutes till light brown. move the chicken to the plate

- Add the remaining one spoonful of oil, carrots, onions, celery, and carrots in the same pot. Cook for five minutes until the vegetables are tender. Add the bay leaf, Garlic, and oregano (1/2 teaspoon) cook for around 30 to 60 seconds,

- Add broth and let it boil over a high flame. Add orzo. Then lower the heat for five minutes to let it simmer, cover, and let it cook. Add the chicken and kale and any leftover juices. Continue cooking for ten minutes until the orzo is soft, and the chicken is cooked through.

- Remove from flame. Throw away the bay leaf; add lemon zest and lemon juice, 3/4 tsp, salt, and 1/4 tsp. of pepper.

Nutrition per serving: Calories 245|Net carbs 20g| protein 12 g|fat12 g| sodium 77 mg

Chapter 11:
Intermittent Fasting Salad & Soups Recipes

11.1 Sauerkraut Salad

(Ready in about: 20 minutes | Serving 6)

Ingredients

- Finely chopped celery: 1 cup

- 1 can of (1 lb.) sauerkraut, do not rinse it but drain it

- 3⁄4 cup of sugar

- 2 tablespoons onions, chopped fine

- Half teaspoon of salt

- Half cup of finely chopped green pepper

- Salad oil: 1⁄3 cup

- Half teaspoon of freshly ground black pepper

- White cider: 1⁄3 cup

Instructions

- In a bowl, add sauerkraut along with chopped up vegetables.

- In a pan, add vinegar, sugar, black pepper, oil, salt on medium flame until sugar dissolves.

- Let it cool and add over chopped up vegetables.

- Let it Chill in the refrigerator overnight.

Nutrition Per serving: 1 out of 6: 224.1 Calories | Cholesterol 0 mg| Sodium 708.5 mg | Total Fat 12.2 g |Total Carbohydrate 29.7 g | Sugars 27.1 g |Protein 1 g| Dietary Fiber 2.8 g |

11.2 Instant Pot Lentil Soup

(Ready in about: 40 minutes | Serving 6)

Ingredients

- Low-sodium vegetable broth: 6 cups

- Olive oil: 2 tbsp.

- Chopped carrots: 1 cup

- Chopped turnip: 1 cup

- Chopped yellow onion: 1 cup

- Thyme: one tbsp.

- Fresh baby spinach: 5 cups

- Brown lentils: 2 cups(washed)

- Salt: ¾ tablespoon

- Radishes: three

- Parsley leaves: ¼ cup

- Balsamic vinegar: 1 and ½ tbsp.

Instructions

- Pick Sauté setting on a multi-cooker programmable pressure.
- Choose High temperature and let it pre-heat.

- Add one tablespoon of oil to a cooker until it becomes hot. Add carrots, onion, thyme, and turnip; fry, frequently stirring, for around 5 minutes, until the onion is tender. Stir in stock, salt, and lentils.

- Select cancel. Let the steam release.

- Before removing the cover from the cooker, stir in vinegar and spinach.

- Toss the parsley and radishes in a wide bowl with the one tablespoon oil.

- Put the soup in six bowls, garnish with radish mixture

Nutrition Per Serving: Calories 305 |total fat 5.5g |carbohydrates 7.5g | protein 18g

11.3 Tomato Green Bean Soup

(Ready in about: 45 minutes| serving 9)

Ingredients

- 4 cups of green beans, fresh, cut into one-inch pieces
- Chopped onion: 1 cup
- Chopped carrots: 1 cup
- Unsalted butter: 2 teaspoons
- Chicken or vegetable low-sodium broth: 6 cups
- Chopped fresh basil: 1/4 cup
- 1 clove of minced garlic
- Chopped fresh tomatoes: 3 cups
- ¼ tsp. of salt
- 1/4 teaspoon of pepper

Instructions

- In a pan, heat the butter, sauté carrots, onions for five minutes. Add in beans, garlic, and broth. Mix it and let it boil. Turn the heat low, cover it, and let it simmer for 20 minutes or till vegetables are soft.

- Add in the salt, tomatoes, basil, pepper. Cover again and let it simmer for five minutes.
- Either puree it or serve it as.
- Enjoy.

Nutrition per cup: Calories 58 | 10g carbohydrate |1g fat |1g saturated fat| | 4g protein |2mg cholesterol|335mg sodium | 4g sugars|3g fiber.

11.4 Turkey & Vegetable Barley Soup

(Ready in about: 30 minutes| Serving 6)

Ingredients

- 1 diced onion
- Canola oil: 1 tablespoon
- Five diced carrots
- Fresh baby spinach: 2 cups
- Quick-cooking barley: 2/3 cup
- Cooked turkey breast: 2 cups, cut into cubes
- Half teaspoon of black pepper
- Chicken broth, reduced-sodium: 6 cups

Instructions

- In a pan, sauté onion and carrots in oil over medium flame for five minutes until tender crispy.
- Add in broth, barley, let it boil. Turn the heat low, let it simmer for 10 to 15 minutes uncovered.
- Add in pepper, turkey, and spinach and; heat it through.
- Serve right away and enjoy

Nutrition per serving: 1-1/3 cups: 208 calories| 23g carbohydrate|4g fat |37mg| cholesterol| 1g saturated fat|462mg sodium| 6g fiber| 21g protein|4g sugars|

11.5 Cobb Salad with Brown Derby Dressing

(Ready in about: 30 minutes| Serving 2)

Ingredients

- 2 tomatoes, medium-sized peeled and removed seeds

- Half head of iceberg lettuce

- One cup of turkey breast, smoked

- One bunch of chicory lettuce

- 6 slices of crisp bacon

- Half head of romaine lettuce

- One avocado, cut in half, peeled, and pit removed

- Half bunch of watercress

- Finely chopped chives: 2 tablespoons

- Half cup of crumbled blue cheese

- Hardboiled egg: three

Dressing

- Water: 2 tablespoons

- Worcestershire sauce: 1⁄2 teaspoon

- Sugar: 1⁄8 teaspoon

- Balsamic vinegar: 2 tablespoons

- Dijon mustard: 1⁄8 teaspoon

- Extra virgin olive oil: 2 tablespoons

- Fresh lemon juice: 1 tablespoon

- 2 cloves of minced garlic

- Kosher salt: 3⁄4 teaspoon

- Fresh ground black pepper: half tsp.

Instructions

- Finely chop the green vegetables very thinly

- In a bowl, add all salad dressing ingredients, mix well in a blender, and set it aside.

- In a chilled bowl of salad, add thinly sliced green vegetables in rows.

- Chop up the tomatoes very thinly.

- Dice the eggs, turkey, bacon, and avocado.

- Add all chopped up ingredients in the bowl, with cheese, in rows.

- Add chives.

- Present like this, toss the salad at eating time, meanwhile, keep in refrigerator to chill as much as possible.

- Serve with croutons, if you like.

- Drizzle dressing over after tossing the salad.

Note: Replace or omit blue cheese if you do not like, or if your main goal is to lose weight.

Nutrition per serving: one of two serving: 832.4 Calories | Cholesterol 352.4 mg| Total Carbohydrate 31.2 g| Total Fat 56.7 g| Sugars 12.4 g| Protein 55 g| Saturated Fat 16.1 g| Dietary Fiber 13.5 g| sodium 460.1 mg|

11.6 Pumpkin Thai Soup

(Ready in about: 65 minutes| Serving 3-4)

Ingredients

- 4 cloves of sliced garlic
- Pumpkin: 2 and a half cusp
- Soy milk: ½ cup
- Extra virgin Olive oil: 1 tablespoon
- Vegetable stock: 3 cups
- Lemongrass: 1 tablespoon (white part), diced
- Two shredded kaffir lime leaves
- One turmeric sliced
- Coriander seeds: 1 teaspoon
- One small red chili de-seeded, thinly sliced
- Cumin seeds: 1 teaspoon
- One onion, diced
- Black pepper
- One-inch ginger minced

Instructions

- Let the oven preheat to 350 F. Add baking paper on a tray.
- Chop the peeled pumpkin, coat with soy milk, and roast until golden.
- In a pot, heat oil, sauté onion till golden, add coriander seeds, cumin
- Cook for a few minutes

- Add garlic, lemongrass, chili, ginger, kaffir leaves, turmeric, cook for another minute. Do not overcook

- Add broth and pumpkin, cover it and let it boil. Let it simmer for t10 minutes. Add milk, increase the heat.

- Cook for 5-10 minutes.

Nutrition per serving: Calories: 349 | Carbohydrates: 35g | Protein: 11g | Fat: 21g | Saturated Fat: 17g | Sodium: 225mg | Fiber: 3g | Sugar: 11g | Calcium: 130mg |

11.7 Beef & Vegetable Soup

(Ready in about: 50 minutes| Serving 4-5)

Ingredients

- Carrots: ½ cup, diced

- 4 cups of beef stew

- Sliced onions: 1 cup

- Basil: ½ tsp

- Green peas: ½ cup

- 3 ½ cup of water

- Black pepper: 1 tsp

- Corn: ½ cup

- Okra: ½ cup

- Thyme: ½ tsp

Instructions

- In a pot, add black pepper, beef stew, water, onions, thyme, and basil

- Cook for 45 minutes.

- Add all vegetables let it simmer on low heat till meat is tender. Enjoy.

Nutrition per serving: Calories 190 | Sodium 56 mg| Protein 11 g| Potassium 291 mg| phosphorus 121 mg| Calcium 31 mg| Fat 13 g| Water 130 g| Carbohydrates 7 g

11.8 Slow Cooker Cabbage Soup

(Ready in about: 8 hours| Serving 4-5)

Ingredients

- Two cloves of minced garlic

- Carrots: 1 cup, diced

- One onion diced

- Cabbage: 4 cups, chopped

- Green beans: 1 cup trimmed into one-inch pieces

- 2 celery stalks diced

- 2 bell peppers diced

- Tomato paste: 2 tablespoons

- 2 bay leaves

- Fresh kale: 2 cups roughly chopped

- Low sodium stock vegetable: 6 cups

- Italian seasoning: 1 and a half tsp.

- Pepper

- Basil: 1 tablespoon

- Parsley: 1 tablespoon

Instructions

- In a pot, add vegetables. Add tomato paste, Italian seasoning, broth, pepper, bay leaves. Mix well

- Cook on high for five hours or slow on 8 hours in a slow cooker.

- After its cooked, add basil, parsley, kale, and cook for five minutes and serve.

Nutrition per serving: Calories: 40|Carbohydrates: 6g| Protein: 2g|Sodium: 64mg| Potassium: 158mg| Fiber: 1g| Sugar: 2g| Calcium: 28mg|Iron: 0.7mg

11.9 Slow Cooker Chicken Rice Soup

(Ready in about: 6-10 hours | Serving 7-8)

Ingredients

- Chicken broth or water: 9 cups

- 6 cups of chicken pieces

- 2 cloves of minced garlic

- 2 cups sliced mushrooms

- Two carrots, roughly chopped

- Cauliflower: one and a half cups

- 3 celery stalks, chopped

- One large onion, finely diced

- Almond milk: 2 cups

- Wild rice: 1 and a half cups

- Mustard: 1 tbsp.

- Garlic powder: 2 tsp

- Ground black pepper, to taste

- Half tsp dried thyme

- 2 tsp of salt

Instructions

- In a slow cooker, add garlic, chicken, celery, onion, carrots, mushrooms, cauliflower, pepper, wild rice, salt, water, and thyme. Cover it and cook for 8-10 hours on Low or for 5-6 hours on High.

- Take chicken out and shred it. in the slow cooker, add garlic powder, milk, and mustard

- Blend the soup and return to the pot.

- Add the shredded chicken, serve hot

Nutrition per serving: Calories 251 | Sodium 123 mg| Protein 13.2 g| Potassium 292 mg| phosphorus 131 mg| Calcium 25.4 mg| Fat 8.9 g| | Carbohydrates 8.6 g

11.10 Chicken Corn Soup

(Ready in about: 40 minutes| Serving 5-6)

Ingredients

- Water: 14 cups

- 4 pound of roasting chicken

- Dried parsley: 1 tablespoon

- Half cups and a little more uncooked flat noodles

- 2 cans of unsalted corn

- Black pepper: 1/4 teaspoon

Instructions

- In a pot, cook chicken in 8 cups of water. Reserve the broth and cooked chicken separately.

- Cook the noodles as per instructions, without salt. Set it aside.

- Take the fat out from chicken broth. Chop the chicken into pieces.

- In a big pot, add 6 cups of broth, 6 cups of water, chopped chicken.

- Add parsley, corns, pepper, cooked noodles. Let it simmer and then serve

Nutrition per serving: Calories 222| Protein 25 g| Carbohydrates 17 g| Fat 6 g| Cholesterol 67 mg| Sodium 240 mg | Calcium 21 mg| Fiber 1.4 g

11.11 Grilled Southwestern Steak Salad

(Ready in about: 45 minutes| serving 4)

Ingredients

- Olive oil: 1 tablespoon

- 3/4 pound of one beef top one inch of thickness, sirloin steak

- 1/4 teaspoon of ground cumin

- Bow tie pasta, uncooked multigrain: 2 cups

- 1/4 teaspoon of freshly ground black pepper

- Three Poblano peppers, cut in halves and seeds removed

- 1/4 teaspoon of sea salt

- 2 large ears, husks removed, sweet corn

- One onion, slice into half-inch rings

- 2 big tomatoes

Dressing

- 1/8 teaspoon of salt

- Olive oil: 1 tablespoon

- 1/4 teaspoon of ground cumin

- Lime juice: 1/4 cup

- Fresh cilantro chopped: 1/3 cup

- 1/4 teaspoon of freshly ground black pepper

Instructions

- Marinate the steak with cumin, pepper, and salt. Toss onion, poblano peppers, onion, and corn with olive oil.

- Grill the steak, cover it over medium flame for 6 to 8 minutes, on each side, until inserted thermometer reads 135 for rare, 140 for medium, and 145 for well-done cooked steak.

- Also, grill the vegetables, cover it for 8 to 10 minutes or till tender, turning halfway through.

- Cook pasta as per instructions, omitting salt. In the meantime, chop roughly the tomatoes, peppers, onion, and cut the cob's corn.

- Add all vegetables to a bowl. In another bowl, mix oil, pepper, salt, lime juice, and cumin. Mix well, then add cilantro.

- Add cooked pasta to vegetables. Pour dressing over. Mix well.

- Cut the cooked steak into slices serve on top of the salad.

- Enjoy.

Nutrition per serving: 2 ounces of cooked beef steak +2 cups of pasta: 456 calories| 30g protein |13g fat|15g sugars|3g saturated fat| 34mg cholesterol| 58g carbohydrate |8g fiber|378mg sodium|

11.12 Strawberry- Cheese Steak Salad

(Ready in about: 30 minutes| serving 4)

Ingredients

- Half teaspoon of salt

- Lime juice: 2 tablespoons

- Freshly ground black pepper: 1/4 teaspoon

- 1 beef top sirloin steak

- Extra virgin olive oil: 2 teaspoons

Salad

- Diced walnuts: 1/4 cup, toasted

- 10 cups of a torn bunch of romaine

- Red onion, thinly sliced: 1/4 cup

- Balsamic vinaigrette, reduced-fat: few tablespoons

- Crumbled feta cheese: 1/4 cup

- Fresh strawberries, 2 cups, sliced in halves

Instructions

- Add pepper, salt to steak. In a skillet, heat the oil, and cook steak for 5 to 7 minutes, brown on every side, until internal temperature reaches 135 F for rare, 145 for well done, and 140 for medium. Cook to your liking.

- Turn off the heat and rest for five minutes. Cut into one-inch pieces and drizzle with lime juice.

- On a serving platter, add romaine on the bottom, top with onion, strawberries, and steak pieces. Add nuts and cheese drizzle with vinaigrette.

- Serve and enjoy.

Nutrition per serving: 289 calories|12g carbohydrate| 4g fiber |15g fat |4g saturated fat| 452mg sodium|52mg cholesterol|5g sugars | 29g protein

11.13 Edamame Salad with Sesame Ginger Dressing

(Ready in about: 15 minutes| serving 6)

Ingredients

- Bean sprouts, fresh: 1 cup

- Baby kale salad mix: 6 cups

- Shelled edamame, frozen: 2 cups must be thawed

- Two green onions, finely sliced

- 3 clementine's, segmented and peeled

- Half cup of unsalted peanuts

- Ginger sesame salad dressing: half cup

- One can of (15 ounces) chickpeas, rinsed, drained

Instructions

- Place salad mix kale in six bowls, add remaining ingredients equally.

- Mix well, add dressing, toss it again

- Serve right away.

Nutrition per serving: one bowl: calories317|32g carbohydrate|17g fat|13g protein |2g saturated fat| 355mg sodium| 0 cholesterol| 14g sugars|8g fiber

11.14 Spinach Orzo Salad with Chickpeas

(Ready in about: 30 minutes| Serving 12)

Ingredients

- 2 cans of (15 ounces each) of chickpeas, rinsed, drained

- One can of (14 and a half ounces) of chicken broth, reduced-sodium

- 1 and a half cups of orzo pasta whole wheat, uncooked

- Grape tomatoes: 2 cups, cut into halves

- 2 diced green onions

- Baby spinach, fresh: 4 cups

- Fresh parsley chopped: 3/4 cup

Dressing

- Lemon juice: 3 tablespoons

- Hot pepper sauce: 1/4 teaspoon

- Salt: 1/4 teaspoon

- Olive oil: 1/4 cup

- Garlic powder: 1/4 teaspoon

- Black pepper: 1/4 teaspoon

Instructions

- In a pot, cook pasta as per instructions, omitting salt.

- In a bowl, add hot pasta, spinach, let the spinach wilt a little. Add green onions, parsley, tomatoes, and chickpeas.

- In a bowl, add all dressing ingredients.

- Pour over salad and toss well.

Nutrition per serving: 3/4 cup: 122 calories| 16g carbohydrate | 4g fiber |5g fat | 259mg |1g saturated fat sodium |1g sugars | 4g protein| 0 g cholesterol

11.15 Zucchini Noodle Salad

(Ready in about: 15 minutes| Serving 4)

Ingredients

- Two zucchinis

- 1 onion peeled

- 2 cloves of crushed garlic

- One cup of bock Choy quarter

- 1 cup: chickpeas

- Red wine vinegar: 2 tablespoons

- Half cup of crumbled feta cheese

- Olive oil: 1/4 cup

- 1 cup of red bell pepper

- Lemon juice: 1 tablespoon

- Dijon mustard: 1 teaspoon

- Salt and pepper to taste

- Dried oregano: 1 teaspoon

Instructions

- In a big jar, add all ingredients and mix.

- Spiralizer the zucchini.

- Spiralizer half the red onion.

- Mix these two noodles

- Add bock Choy, chickpeas, feta cheese in the bowl.

- Add the dressing over vegetables and mix.

- Pour dressing over salad, gently mix everything.

- Serve & enjoy.

Nutrition per serving: Calories: 151 g| Protein: 7.8 g| Carbohydrates: 12.1 g| Fiber: 3.4 g| Total Fat: 2.9 g| Sodium: 103 mg| Phosphorus: 87 mg| Potassium: 92 mg|

11.16 Grilled Chicken Salad with Fig Balsamic Vinaigrette

(Ready in about: 10 minutes| Serving 4)

Ingredients

For the dressing

- Olive oil: ¼ cup

- Dried figs: ¼ cup

- Chopped basil: 2 tablespoons

- Half cup of balsamic vinegar

- Salt, a pinch

- Pepper, to taste

- Lemon zest: 1 teaspoon

For the salad

- Pea shoots: ¼ cup

- One radish, cut into thin slices

- ¼ cup of diced grilled chicken breast

- Half medium pear, cut into thin slices

Instructions

- In a blender, add olive oil, figs, balsamic vinegar, pulse until smooth.

- Add lemon zest, basil. Season with pepper, salt to taste. Mix it well and set it aside.

- Add radishes, pears, pea shoots, and arugula in that order. Seal and refrigerate.

- In a bowl, add chicken breast, pour dressing over, and serve.

Nutrition Per Serving: 224 calories| sugar 11g| total fat 15g| sodium 172mg| fiber 2g| carbohydrates 14g| saturated fat 2g| protein 9g

11.17 Yellow Pear & Cherry Tomato Salad

(Ready in about: 15 minutes| serving 6)

Ingredients

- Extra-virgin olive oil: 1 tablespoon

- Minced onion: 1 tablespoon

- 1 and a half cups of red cherry tomatoes, cut into halves

- Salt: 1/4 teaspoon

- Red wine vinegar: 2 tablespoons

- Freshly ground black pepper: 1/8 teaspoon

- 1 and a half cups of cherry orange tomatoes, cut into halves

- Fresh basil leaves: 4 large, slice into thin ribbons

- 1 and a half cups of yellow pear tomatoes, cut into halves

Instructions

- In a bowl, mix onion and vinegar. Let it rest for 15 minutes.
- Add salt, olive oil, and pepper and mix until smooth.
- In a big bowl, add all tomatoes, pour vinaigrette over, add basil and mix well.
- Serve it right away.

Nutrition per serving: ¾ cup of salad: Calories 47| Total fat 3 g| Protein 1 g| Cholesterol 0 mg| Total carbohydrate 4 g| Dietary fiber 1 g | sodium 13 mg|

11.18 Mix Vegetable Soup

(Ready in about: 30 minutes| Serving 3-4)

Ingredients

- Two extra virgin olive oil teaspoons
- 1 and ½ carrot cups, shredded
- Six cloves of garlic, minced
- 1 cup of yellow, chopped onion
- 1 cup of diced celery
- Low-sodium chicken stock: 4 cups
- Four Cups of Water
- 1 and ½ cups pasta
- Two tablespoons of parsley
- ¼ cup low-fat, grated parmesan

Instructions

- Over medium-high warm, warm a pan with the oil, add garlic, mix and simmer for 1 minute.
- Add the onion, celery, and carrot, stir, and roast for 7 minutes.
- Add onion, water and pasta, stir, bring to a boil, and simmer for Eight more minutes over moderate flame.
- Split into cups, top, and serve each with parsley and parmesan.

Nutrition per serving: calories 212| fat 4 g| fiber 4 g| carbs 13 g| protein 8 g| potassium 198 mg| phosphorous 109 mg

Chapter 12:

Intermittent Fasting Fish & Seafood Recipes

12.1 Fish Tacos with Cumin Sour Cream & Broccoli Slaw

(Ready in about: 15 minutes| Serving 4)

Ingredients

- Eight tortillas

- Low sodium Fish sticks: 2 10-oz. Packages

- Half red onion sliced

- Two limes, juiced and wedges

- Broccoli: 12 ounces

- Kosher salt: 1 tsp.

- Olive oil: 2 tablespoons

- Half cup of low-fat, sour cream

- Cilantro: 1 cup

- Half tsp. of ground cumin

Instructions

- According to the direction on the package, cook the fish sticks.

- Chop broccoli' heads. Peel the stalks and cut them into matchsticks.

- In a large bowl, add the lime juice, onion, and 3/4 teaspoon of salt.; mix and set aside around ten minutes.

- Add broccoli stalks and tops, oil, cilantro, and mix

- Mix cumin, sour cream, and salt in a small dish. Serve with fish

Nutrition Per Serving: 227 calories| total fat 14 g | carbohydrates 12.5 g| protein 20.3 g | Cholesterol 7.1 mg| Sodium 120 mg| potassium 109 mg| Phosphorus 102 mg |Calcium 6.1 mg| Fiber 3 g

12.2 Baked Fish with Mushrooms & Roasted Sweet Potatoes

(Ready in about: 50 minutes| Serving 4)

Ingredients

- Wild Salmon: 1 and ½ cup, cut into four pieces

- Sweet potatoes cubed: 2 cups, leached

- Olive oil divided: two tbsp.

- Salt: ¼ tsp.

- Herbs: 1 tsp.

- Mushrooms: 4 cups(sliced)

- Two cloves garlic: sliced

- Lemon juice: 4 tbsp.

- Ground pepper: ¼ tsp.

- Thyme

Instructions

- Let the oven heat till 425 F

- Add one tbsp. of oil, potatoes, mushroom, pepper, and salt in a bowl.

- Transfer it to a baking dish and roast for almost forty minutes until the vegetables are soft. Stir the vegetables and add. garlic

- Place fish over it. Drizzle with one tbsp. of oil, lemon juice. Sprinkle with herbs bake till fish is flaky for fifteen minutes.

Nutrition Per Serving: 275 calories| total fat 16.8 g | carbohydrates 15.4 g| protein 21.3 g | Cholesterol 5.3 mg| Sodium 132 mg| Calcium 56 mg| Fiber 2.3 g

12.3 Salmon Cakes

(Ready in about: 30 minutes| Serving 4)

Ingredients

- One tablespoon of olive oil
- Garlic (minced): 1/2 tsp
- Salmon: 5 oz. cooked and finely diced
- Smoked paprika: 1/4 tsp
- 3 - 4 tablespoon of flour
- Fine kosher or sea salt: 1/4 tsp
- Curry powder: 1/4 tsp (optional)
- One sprig of rosemary
- Black pepper: 1/4 tsp
- Two egg whites

Instructions

- Mashup the salmon. remove any skin, if any
- Put the salmon in a bowl, then add the mashed veggies.
- Then add one tbsp. at a time in flour. Depending on the kind of salmon you choose, you'll need just 3-4 tbsp. Then add in herbs and seasonings. Mix well.
- Finally, add in two eggs.

- Mix well that the batter gets thick enough for patties to shape. Add one tbsp. More flour if the batter is too liquid.

- Shape into small or larger balls. then turn them into patties

- Turn the skillet on to medium flame, add butter

- When hot, put in at least three or four cakes at a time. Cook on either side for almost four minutes, or until the salmon is fully cooked. Canned salmon cooks early; repeat the frying process for the rest of the cakes.

- Garnish with black pepper, rosemary, chili flakes, and a sprinkle of garlic if needed, serve hot.

Nutrition Per Serving: 91 calories| total fat 4 g | carbohydrates 6 g| protein 10 g | Cholesterol 4.3 mg| Sodium 101 mg| Calcium 33 mg| Fiber 2.8 g

12.4 Salmon Parcels with Pesto, & Broccoli

(Ready in about: 40 minutes| Serving 2)

Ingredients

- Salmon fillets: one cup

- Rice: one cup

- Red pesto: 3 tablespoon

- One lemon: half juiced and half thinly sliced

- Purple sprouting broccoli: half cup

- Black olives chopped: 2 tablespoon

- Basil

Instructions

- Let the overheat till 200 C to gas6, a 180 C. line the baking tray with parchment paper. Separate the mixed grains and rice. Stir in the lemon juice, olives, 2 tbsp. of pesto and half of the basil. Mix well, put in the center of the baking tray

- Place the salmon over the grains and scatter over each fillet the remaining pesto. Cover with the slices of lemon and broccoli, then cover with parchment paper on top. make it a packet around filling

- Roast for about half an hour in the oven till broccoli is soft and salmon is completely cooked

- Serve with basil on top.

Nutrition Per Serving: 361 calories| total fat 16.2 g | carbohydrates 18 g| protein 9 g | Cholesterol 5.1 mg| Sodium 114 mg| potassium 121 mg| Phosphorus 109 mg |Calcium 56 mg| Fiber 3.2 g

12.5 Swordfish with Capers, & Olives

(Ready in about: 40 minutes| Serving 4)

Ingredients

- Chopped red peppers: 2 Cups

- Half cup of regular or coarse yellow cornmeal

- Swordfish: 4 cups, cut into four steaks

- 2 and ½ cups of water

- Extra-virgin olive oil: 1 tablespoon

- Chopped fresh basil: 3 tablespoons

- 4 medium stalks celery, chopped

- ¼ of cup green olives pitted and roughly diced

- Capers: 1 tablespoon rinsed

- A pinch of crushed red pepper

- Half teaspoon of salt, divided

- 2 cloves of pressed garlic

- For garnish Fresh basil

- Freshly ground black pepper: ⅛ teaspoon

Instructions

- Put a saucepan over medium flame and boil two cups of water with 1/4 tsp. of salt. Add the cornmeal carefully to avoid any lumps.

- Cook for three minutes; keep stirring.

- Lower the heat. Stir after every five minutes, cook for 20-25 minutes. If it becomes too hard, add a half cup of water, turn off the heat but keep it covered.

- In the meantime, in a large skillet over a medium flame, add in the oil. Add celery fry it, frequently stirring, until soft, for around five minutes.

- Then add garlic, cook for almost 30 seconds. Add in olives, bell peppers, basil, crushed red pepper, capers, freshly ground black pepper, and the remaining 1/4 tsp. of Sea salt.

- Cover it lower the heat, and cook for five minutes.

- Add swordfish to the sauce. Let it simmer, and Cover it cook for 10-15 minutes, till swordfish is cooked completely.

- On a serving tray, layer the cornmeal at the bottom. Add the fish over the cornmeal, cover with the sauce and, garnish with fresh basil; serve hot and enjoy.

Nutrition Per Serving: 276 calories| total fat 12.1 g | carbohydrates 13.2 g| protein 22 g | Cholesterol 5.3 mg| Sodium 131 mg| Calcium 46 mg| Fiber 2.4 g

12.6 Roasted Fish with Vegetables

(Ready in about: 15 minutes| Serving 2-3)

Ingredients

- Four skinless salmon fillets: 5-6 ounces

- Two red, yellow, orange sweet peppers, cut into rings

- Five cloves of garlic chopped

- Sea salt: half tsp.

- Olive oil: 2 tbsp.

- Black pepper: half tsp

- Pitted halved olives: ¼ cup

- One lemon

- Parsley: 1 and ½ cups

- Finely snipped fresh oregano:1/4 cup

Instructions

- Let the oven preheat to 425 F

- Put the potatoes in a bowl. Drizzle 1 spoon of oil, sprinkle with salt (1/8 tsp.), and garlic. Mix well, shift to the baking pan, cover with foil. Roast them for half an hour

- In the meantime, thaw the salmon. Combine the sweet peppers, parsley, oregano, olives, salt (1/8 tsp) and pepper in the same bowl. Add one tablespoon of oil, mix well.

- Wash salmon and dry it with paper towels. Sprinkle with salt (1/4 Tsp), Black pepper, and top of it, salmon. Uncover it and roast for ten minutes or till salmon starts to flake.

- Add lemon zest and lemon juice over salmon and vegetables. Serve hot

Nutrition Per Serving: 278 calories| total fat 12 g | carbohydrates 9.2 g| protein 15.4 g | Cholesterol 7.1 mg| Sodium 131 mg| potassium 141 mg| Phosphorus 121 mg

12.7 Salmon with Brussel Sprout

(Ready in about: 15 minutes| Serving 2)

Ingredients

- Steamed Brussels: 1 cup

- Fresh salmon: 4 ounces

- Light soy sauce: 2 tablespoons

- Dijon mustard: 1 and 1/2 tablespoons

- Salt & pepper, to taste

Instructions

- Let the broiler pre-heat. Cover the salmon surface with mustard and soy sauce.

- Spray the baking sheet with oil, put salmon in the baking pan, and broil for ten minutes, or until salmon is completely cooked through.

- Meanwhile, steam the Brussel sprout, if not already steamed

- Serve salmon and sprinkle salt & pepper to taste.

Nutrition per serving: Calories 236|Protein 15.3 g |Carbohydrates 7.2 g| Fat 16.4 g| Cholesterol 8.9 mg| Sodium 143 mg| potassium 176 mg| Phosphorus 132 mg

12.8 Charred Shrimp & Pesto Buddha Bowls

(Ready in about: 15 minutes| Serving 4)

Ingredients

- Pesto: 1/3 cup

- Vinegar: 2 tbsp.

- Olive oil: 1 tbsp.

- Salt: 1/8 tsp.

- Ground pepper: ¼ tsp.

- Peeled & deveined large shrimp: one pound

- Arugula: 4 cups

- Cooked quinoa: 2 cups

Instructions

- In a large bowl, mix pesto, oil, vinegar, salt, and pepper. Take out four tbsp. of mixture in another bowl.

- Place skillet over medium flame. Add shrimp, let it cook for five minutes, stirring, until only charred a little. move to a plate

- Use the vinaigrette to mix with quinoa and arugula in a bowl. Divide the mixture of the arugula into four bowls. Cover with shrimp, add 1 tbsp. of the pesto mixture to each bowl, and serve.

Nutrition Per Serving: 329 calories| total fat 18 g | carbohydrates 17.2 g| protein 17 g | Cholesterol 6.7 mg| Sodium 154 mg| potassium 143 mg| Phosphorus 123 mg

12.9 Cilantro-Lime Swordfish

(Ready in about: 15 minutes| Serving 2-3)

Ingredients

- Swordfish: 1 pound

- Half cup of low-fat mayonnaise

- Lime juice: 2 tablespoon

- Half cup of fresh cilantro

Instructions

- In a bowl, mix chopped cilantro, lime juice, low-fat mayonnaise, mix well.

- Take ¼ cup from the mix and leave the rest aside

- Apply the rest of the mayo mix to the fish with a brush

- In a skillet, over medium heat, spray oil

- Add fish fillets, cook for 8 minutes, turning once, or until fish is cooked to your liking.

- Serve with sauce.

Nutrition per serving: Calories 292 | Protein 20 g |Carbohydrates 1 g| Fat 23 g| Cholesterol 57 mg| Sodium 228 mg| Potassium 237 mg| Phosphorus 128 mg

12.10 Pesto-Crusted Catfish

(Ready in about: 25 minutes| Serving 4)

Ingredients

- Pesto: 4 teaspoons

- Catfish: 2 pounds (no bones)

- Panko bread crumbs: ¾ cup

- Olive oil: 2 tablespoons

- Half cup of vegan cheese

- Seasoning Blend: (No salt added spices)

- Red pepper flakes: half teaspoon

- Garlic powder, low sodium: 1 teaspoon

- Dried oregano: half teaspoon

- Black pepper: half teaspoon

- Onion powder: 1 teaspoon

Instructions

- Let the oven preheat to 400 F

- In a bowl, add all the seasoning, sprinkle over fish on both sides.

- Then spread pesto on each side of fish

- In a bowl, mix bread crumbs, cheese, oil—coat pesto fish in crumbs mix.

- Spray oil on the baking tray. Add fish on a baking tray.

- Bake at 400° F for 20 minutes or until it's ready.

- Let it rest for ten minutes. Then serve.

Nutrition Per Serving: Calories 312 | total Fat 16 g | Cholesterol 83 mg| Sodium 272 mg| Carbohydrates 15 g| Protein 26 g| Phosphorus 417 mg| Potassium 576 mg|

12.11 Citrusy Salmon

(Ready in about: 20 minutes| Serving 4)

Ingredients

- Salmon filet: 24 ounces/3 cups

- Olive oil: 2 tablespoons

- Dijon mustard: 1 tablespoon

- Two garlic cloves, minced

- Dried basil leaves: 1 teaspoon

- Lemon juice: 1-1/2 tbsp.

- Unsalted butter: 1 tablespoon

- Cayenne pepper: 2 pinches

- Capers: 1 tablespoon

- Dried dill: 1 teaspoon

Instructions

- In a pan, add all the ingredients but do not add salmon. Let it boil, then lower the flame and cook for five minutes.

- Preheat the grill. Put the fish on a large piece of foil, skin side down.

- Fold the edges. Put the fish in foil on the grill. Add sauce over the salmon.

- Cover the grill, let it cook for 12 minutes, do not flip the fish.

- Serve hot.

Nutrition per serving: Calories 294| Protein 23 g| Carbohydrates 1 g| Fat 22 g| Cholesterol 68 mg| Sodium 190 mg| Potassium 439 mg| Phosphorus 280 mg

12.12 Oven-Fried Cod with Avocado Puree Recipe

(Ready in about : 30 minutes | Serving 4)

Ingredients

- One avocado: chopped
- Cod filets: 4 6-ounce
- (Powder) cornmeal: ¼ cup
- Half cup minced red onion
- Lime juice: 2 tablespoons
- Salt and black pepper: ¼ teaspoon each

Instructions

- Let the oven pre-heat to 400 F and spray with oil generously. Blend salt and pepper with cornmeal.
- Dip the fish into the cornmeal blend gently. Put on the baking sheet. Drizzle olive oil on top of tuna, then put it in the oven.
- Bake for 20 minutes till it is cooked.
- Mix the mashed avocado with the salt, red onion, and lime juice,
- Serve a big spoon of avocado puree with the fish.

Nutrition Per Serving: 131 calories|6g fat |11g carbs |9g protein| fiber 0.8 g| sodium 34 mg

Conclusion

Intermittent fasting or IF, often referred to as intermittent energy restriction, is a generic word for specific meal timing schedules that exist over a specified time of voluntary non-fasting and fasting.

The clinical literature reviews appeared to have nothing bad to tell about the drawback of intermittent fasting for women over 50 other than suggesting that potential benefits are many. Intermittent fasting is safe for pre and post-menopausal women.

These are the more highlighted benefits of intermittent fasting for post-menopausal women.

- **Losing weight**: Intermittent fasting will help you shed extra pounds and belly fat without needing to ration calories, as described above deliberately. Insulin sensitivity: intermittent fasting will decrease insulin resistance and reduce blood sugar by 3 to percent, and it will help in type 2 diabetes
- **Reduction in Inflammation**: Several reports indicate declines in inflammation markers, a primary driver of many chronic illnesses.
- **Healthy Heart:** Poor LDL cholesterol, inflammation receptors, blood triglycerides, insulin tolerance, blood sugar, and maybe decreased through intermittent fasting; these are risk factors for heart failure.
- **Low risk of Cancer:** Studies in mammals indicate that intermittent fasting can lower the risk of cancer.
- **Healthy Brain**: Intermittent fasting raises the BDNF, a brain hormone, and can help the development of new nerve cells. It can guard against Alzheimer's disease as well.
- **Anti-aging:** IF in mammals will prolong life expectancy. Studies have shown that 36 to 83 percent of fasted mammals live longer

Intermittent fasting is not a magical way for weight reduction that works for everyone, but it does not work for everybody. Some individuals consider it might not be as effective for women as men, but results have proven otherwise. It is often not advised to practice intermittent fasting for those who have or are susceptible to eating disorders.

Bear in mind the diet's consistency is important if you plan to pursue intermittent fasting. It is not realistic to gorge on fatty foods during feeding time and hopes to lose weight and improve your fitness. Note that food and calorie consistency are always really necessary and cannot be overlooked, regardless of what intermittent fasting one plans to adopt. Sometimes, when they utilize intermittent fasting as a protective net, individuals may side-line food consistency or overindulge in calories. This will not be successful in the long term, and your well-being will be affected.

To know which fasting style you like better, have fun, and try multiple intermittent fasting ways.

INTERMITTENT FASTING 16/8

The Ultimate Step-By-Step Guide To 8-Hour Diet, Which Makes You Live Healthy, Lose Weight, Burn Fat and Age Slowly with Autophagy and Metabolism, Including Recipes

By

Asuka Young

Introduction

Intermittent Fasting (IF) is known to be the dietary eating patterns, which include a prolonged period of not eating or severely restricting calories. There are many different intermittent fasting subgroups, each with individual differences in the length of the fast; some for hours, some for day(s). This has become a prevalent subject within the scientific community due to all the potential benefits that are being found in terms of fitness and safety.

There are no excuses for not moving. People often think they have no other option than to keep gaining weight, but maintaining the ideal weight is essential for health. Even losing weight in the right way is equally important.

Being overweight or clinically obese means having a high caloric intake and low energy expenditure. To lose weight, it is important to reduce calorie intake both with the diet and by practicing regular physical activity because the diet is always more effective when combined with movement. In any case, combining physical activity makes the diet more and more effective.

Many people work out to lose weight, but they do it the wrong way because they think that intense cardio exercise or prolonged sessions allow them to lose weight faster and keep the extra pounds away. This method actually turns out to be ineffective. In order not to lose the benefits of training, it is important to watch your diet more closely.

A widespread habit among those who want to lose weight is to practice fasting. If on one hand, it can be an advantage, on the other it is risky for health. The recommended duration of fasting aerobic activity is about 40 minutes; beyond this duration, it is possible to resort to the consumption of stock proteins, with consequent muscle catabolism, that is, destruction of muscle mass.

It is natural to reduce the amount of food taken to decrease calorie intake. However, adopting a regulated food intake, such as diets based only on the consumption of fruit and vegetables and eliminating certain foods altogether has been proven more effective than other methods of weight loss. In this cookbook, we present recipes, which can make you lose weight pretty fast and more effectively without any form of side effect.

Physical activity and nutrition are two main complementary elements. To lose weight intelligently, you need to combine the right amount of physical activity with a correct diet.

Chapter 1:
What Is Intermittent Fasting (IF)?

Intermittent fasting (IF) is the pattern of eating, which cycles between fasting and eating periods. It does not dictate what foods to consume, but rather when to eat. It's not a diet in a conventional manner, but more accurately described as a method of eating in this way.

Common methods of intermittent fasting involve 16-hour daily fasts or 24-hour fasting, twice a week. Fasting was a practice throughout all of human evolution. Ancient hunter-gatherers didn't have all-year-round supermarkets, refrigerators, or milk. They were sometimes unable to find anything to cook.

As a consequence, humans evolved to be able to function for extended periods without food. It is more natural to fast regularly than always eating 3–4 (or more) meals a day. Fasting is also often carried out for religious or spiritual purposes, in Islam, Christianity, Judaism, and Buddhism, among others.

Intermittent Fasting Methods

There are several ways to do intermittent fasting— all of which involve splitting the day or week into periods of eating and fasting.During the periods of fasting, you either eat very little or nothing.

Those methods are the most popular:

The 16/8 method: It is often known as the Leangains protocol, which involves skipping breakfast and restricting the average meal time to 8 hours, such as 1–9 pm. Then you'll fast in between for 16 hours.

Eat-Stop-Eat: It includes a 24-hour fast, once or twice a week, e.g., by not eating dinner one day and fasting till the dinner of the next day.

The 5:2 diet: With these approaches, on two non-consecutive days of the week, you consume just 500–600 calories but normally eat the other five days. By lowering the intake of calories, all of these strategies will cause weight loss as long as you don't compensate by eating any more during the feeding time. The 16/8 approach is considered by many to be the most straightforward, most effective, and easy to adhere to. It is the most common one, too.

How It Affects Your Cells and Hormones

When you abstain from eating, many things happen in your body both on the cellular and molecular level. As an example, the body adjusts the hormonal levels to make it more accessible to accumulated body fat. Often, the cells start critical mechanisms of restoring and altering gene expression.

Here are some changes happening in your body when you're fasting:

Human Growth Hormone (HGH): Growth hormone levels surge, rising as much as 5-fold. This has advantages in terms of fat loss and muscle gain, to name a few.

Insulin: Insulin sensitivity increases and insulin levels drop dramatically. Higher insulin levels improve the sensitivity of retained body fat.

Cellular repair: The cells start cellular reparation processes when they fast. This involves autophagy, in which cells digest and remove old and damaged proteins that develop within cells.

Gene expression: There are variations in gene expression associated with survival and disease prevention. Such changes in hormone levels, cell function, and gene expression are responsible for intermittent fasting's health benefits.

A Very Powerful Weight Loss Tool

Weight loss is the most prominent reason people seek intermittent fasting. IF can lead to an automatic reduction in calorie intake by making you eat fewer meals. Intermittent fasting adjusts the rates of the hormones that promote weight loss. It increases the production of the fat-burning hormone norepinephrine (noradrenaline) in addition to reducing insulin and raising growth hormone levels.

Because of these hormone changes, the metabolic rate can be raised by 3.6–14 percent in the short term. Intermittent fasting promotes weight loss by shifting all sides of the calorie equation and making you eat less and burn more calories. Studies have shown intermittent fasting can be a powerful tool for weight loss.

A 2014 research study found that this style of eating would cause weight loss of 3–8 percent over 3–24 weeks, which is a significant amount relative to most studies of weight loss. Participants have lost 4–7 percent of their waist circumference, suggesting a significant loss of unhealthy belly fat that develops around the organs and causes disease, according to the same report.

The study showed that intermittent fasting produces less loss of muscle than the more standard method of daily restriction of calories.

Keep in mind, however, that the main reason for their popularity is that intermittent fasting makes you eat fewer overall calories. If you binge during eating periods and eat massive amounts, you may not lose any weight at all.

Health Benefits

There have been many reports on intermittent fasting in animals as well as in humans. Such findings have shown that it can have significant benefits on your body and brain for weight control and wellbeing. It can even make you go on living longer.

Here are the most significant health effects of intermittent fasting:

Weight loss: As described above, intermittent fasting will help you lose weight and fat on your butt, without deliberately restricting calories.

Insulin resistance: IF can reduce insulin resistance, lower blood sugar by 3–6 percent, and fast insulin levels by 20–31 percent, which should protect against type 2 diabetes.

Inflammation: Several studies show decreases in inflammatory levels, which are a vital driver of many chronic diseases.

Heart health: Intermittent fasting will decrease "poor" LDL cholesterol, triglycerides in the blood, inflammatory markers, blood sugar, and tolerance to insulin— all risk factors for heart disease.

Cancer: Studies show that intermittent fasting also prevents cancer.

Brain health: Intermittent fasting raises the BDNF brain hormone and may help new nerve cells to grow. It could also guard against the condition of Alzheimer's.

Anti-aging: Intermittent fasting can prolong the rat lifespan. Research has shown that fasted rats live longer than 36–83 percent of non-fasted rats.

Remember, research is still in its early stages. Many of the experiments have been small, short-term, or carried out in livestock. For higher quality human studies, several questions are yet to be resolved.

Chapter 2:
16/8 Intermittent Fasting

For thousands of years, fasts have been practiced and are a tradition across many diverse religions and cultures around the world.

Today, modern fasting variations put a new spin on the old practice.

16/8: One of the most popular styles of fasting is intermittent fasting. Proponents claim that weight loss and overall health improvements are an easy, convenient and sustainable way to do so.

This chapter reviews intermittent fasting on 16/8, how it works, and if it's right for you.

What Is 16/8 Intermittent Fasting?

16/8 Intermittent fasting means restricting the consumption of food and calorie-containing drinks to a fixed eight-hour window per day and abstaining from the remainder of the 16 hours from eating.

Depending on your personal choice, this process can be repeated as often as you like — from just once or twice a week to every day.

In recent years, 16/8 intermittent fasting has skyrocketed in popularity, especially among those looking to lose weight and burn fat.

While other diets also set strict rules and regulations, intermittent 16/8 fasting is easy to follow and can provide minimal effort to produce real results.

It is generally regarded as less rigid and more flexible than many other diet plans, and can easily fit into almost any lifestyle.

In addition to enhancing weight loss, it is also believed that 16/8 intermittent fasting will improve blood sugar, boost brain function and improve longevity.

How to Get Started

16/8 Simple, safe and sustainable intermittent fasts.

To get started, first pick an eight-hour window and limit your food intake to that period.

Most people prefer to eat between midday and 8 p.m., as this means that you only need to run overnight and skip breakfast, but you can still eat a balanced lunch and dinner and a few snacks all day long.

Many tend to eat at 9 a.m. Then 5 p.m., leaving plenty of time for a healthy breakfast at 9 a.m., a regular lunch at midday and a light early dinner or snack at 4 p.m.

Before starting your fast, you should experiment with and pick the time frame that best fits your schedule.

Everything you eat, it's recommended that you eat multiple small meals and snacks evenly spaced all day long to help stabilize blood sugar levels and keep appetite under control.

Additionally, it is essential to stick to nutritious whole foods and beverages during your eating periods to maximize diet potential health benefits.

Filling in foods that are rich in nutrients can help you complete your diet and enable you to reap the rewards this diet has to offer.

Try balancing each meal with a tasty variety of whole, healthy foods, like:

Fruits, e.g. apples, bananas, berries, oranges, peaches, pears, etc.

Veggies, e.g. broccoli, cauliflower, cucumbers, leafy greens, tomatoes, etc.

Whole grains, e.g. quinoa, rice, oats, barley, buckwheat, etc.

Healthy fats, e.g. Olive oil

Sources of proteins, e.g. meat, poultry, fish, legumes, eggs, nuts, seeds, etc.

Drinking calorie-free drinks, such as water and unsweetened tea and coffee, can also help control your appetite while keeping you hydrated even while fasting.

Also, binging or overdoing it on junk food can negate the positive effects of 16/8 intermittent fasting and can end up doing more harm to your health than good.

Benefits of 16/8 Intermittent Fasting

16/8 Intermittent fasting is an everyday diet because it is easy to follow, versatile and long-term sustainable.

It's also easy, as it can cut down on how much time and money you need to spend each week on cooking and preparing food.

16/8 intermittent fasting has been linked to a long list of benefits in terms of health, including:

Increased weight loss: Not only does it help to cut calories for the day by restricting the intake to a few hours a day, but also it could boost metabolism and weight loss, studies have revealed.

Improved blood sugar: Intermittent fasting has been shown to reduce the risk of diabetes by up to 31 percent and lower blood sugar by 3–6 percent.

Enhanced longevity: Although evidence in humans is limited, some animal studies have found that longevity may be extended by intermittent fasting.

Is 16/8 Intermittent Fasting Right for Me?

16/8 Intermittent fasting in combination with a nutritious diet and a healthy lifestyle can be a sustainable, safe and easy way to improve your health.

It should not, however, be seen as a replacement for a healthy, well-rounded diet rich in whole foods. Not to mention, even if intermittent fasting isn't working for you, you can still be healthy.

Although intermittent fasting of 16/8 is generally considered safe for most healthy adults, you should speak with your doctor before trying it, especially if you have any underlying health conditions.

This is critical if you take any medications or have asthma, low blood pressure or a history of eating disorders.

IF is also not recommended for women who try to conceive, or get pregnant or breastfeeding women.

Always consult your doctor if you have any concerns or experience any adverse side effects while fasting.

Summary

16/8 Intermittent fasting involves eating only for 8 hours and fasting for the remaining 16 hours.

It can facilitate weight loss and improve blood sugar, brain function and lifespan.

During your mealtime, eat a healthy diet and drink calorie-free drinks such as water or unsweetened teas and coffee.

 Before embarking on intermittent fasting, it is best to speak with your doctor, particularly if you have any underlying health problems.

Chapter 3:
Is 16:8 Fasting Good For Weight Loss?

Different studies have found that there is virtually no difference between people who observed intermittent fasting regularly and those who cut back their overall calorie intake.

A developing body of research shows that a better strategy is to optimize the nutritional rate of what has been eaten (veggies, fruit, lean protein, whole grains, and healthy fats), as opposed to fasting or calorie counting. Science also shows that any potential benefit from fasting is easily lost during the cycle's feeding phase, where appetite-suppressing hormones switch gears and make you feel even hungrier than you did at baseline.

But some dietitians may benefit from day-to-day fasting if they have difficulty adhering to prescribed meal plans; a 2018 pilot study published in the Journal of Nutrition and Safe Eating shows that a 16:8 fasting program may help obese dietitians lose weight by counting every single calorie they consume. This fasting approach might also help those struggling with other weight-related issues— high blood pressure, in particular. A recent academic analysis published in the New England Journal of Medicine indicates that a 16:8 fasting strategy may help the body to naturally improve the control of blood sugar, as well as reduce overall blood pressure over the long term.

Is fasting 16 hours a day healthy?

Intermittent fasting forms such as the 16:8 diet rely on the concept that fasting reduces oxidative stress on the body, which can reduce inflammation and chronic disease risk.

It's also theorized that, according to a recent study published in Cell Metabolism, fasting gives the important organs, digestive and absorptive hormones, and metabolic functions a "break". Since our bodies secrete insulin to help our cells absorb sugar, over time, fasting is associated with reducing our susceptibility to insulin resistance. (In the end, high levels of insulin put us at risk for a whole host of diseases.) However, research also linked fasting with increases in LDL cholesterol (the "bad" type). Intermittent fasting can cause you to feel dizzy and nauseous and cause low blood sugar and dehydration periods. Although most 16:8 enthusiasts drink water during periods of fasting, it may not be enough (remember: the food itself provides quite a bit of water).

I am also much more concerned about the disordered eating behaviors that may arise as a result of intermittent fasting. Research shows that fasting for a period followed by a limited eating prime window gives you an overeat. It's a path that can be difficult to get out of because it impairs the natural hunger signals and metabolism of our body. Limited eating can also cause an increased risk of depression and anxiety.

This is particularly worrying for women, who historically were more likely to develop eating disorders. The allotted restriction periods followed by eating lend themselves to the tendencies of binge-purging that cannot (and should not) be ignored. Periods of vomiting and binging are considered risk factors for eating disorders, according to the National Eating Disorders Association.

Should you try 16:8 fasting?

It's a personal choice, in the end. But you can try some beneficial behaviors without committing to the riskier elements of 16-hour fasts. The first is to understand better the mindfulness of your food choices and how they relate to it. To begin with, put into consideration these questions when deciding on what to take:

Where are you physically when you want to eat?

Many of us feed according to situation, not greed. Case in point: if you ever went to the cinema after dinner, and suddenly wanted popcorn, raise your hand? Yeah, so do I!

You may become mindful of trends you didn't notice before by noticing the moments that you feed. Say that during The Bachelor, you are a person who loves to graze. If you're fasting at 8 p.m., you've automatically cut your post-dinner snacking hours — and then calories— short.

Are you getting enough sleep?

When you cut out snacking late-night, that alone could help you get to bed earlier— a very crucial component of any weight loss plan. Getting seven hours of sleep per night has been linked to better weight management, lowering chronic disease risk and improving metabolism.

For many of us, eliminating food to fixed periods is not feasible to achieve better health. Besides being socially challenging (who wants to skip the happy hour or dinner with friends?), self-imposed rules aren't as satisfied as having the right information and making choices that empower you versus hold you back. In the context of your daily life, it is best to find ways to make eating nutritious food work for you.

Chapter 4:
Popular Ways to Do Intermittent Fasting

Recent years have seen intermittent fasting being very trendy. It is claimed to be causing weight loss, improving metabolic health, and maybe even extending lifespan. Given the popularity, it is not shocking that several different types or methods of intermittent fasting were developed. Every method can be useful, but it depends on the individual to figure out which one works best.

Here are five standard methods to follow intermittent fasting.

1. The 16/8 Method: Fast for 16 hours each day

The 16/8 method involves fasting for 14 to 16 hours every day, and limiting your daily "eating window" to 8-10 hours. You can fit in 2, 3, or more meals within the eating window. Often known as the Leangains Protocol, this approach has been popularized by fitness expert Martin Berkhan. Merely doing this fasting process can be as easy as not eating anything after dinner and skipping breakfast. When you finish your last meal at 8 p.m., for starters, and don't eat before noon the next day, you have been fasting for 16 hours, theoretically.

It is generally recommended that women fast just 14-15 hours because, with significantly shorter fasts, they seem to do well. This approach may be hard to get used to at first for people who are getting hungry in the morning and like to eat breakfast. A lot of breakfast-skippers eat this way instinctively, though. During the fast, you can drink water, coffee, and other non-caloric drinks, which can help to reduce hunger feelings. Mostly eating healthy foods is very important during your feeding time. This method won't work if you're eating lots of junk food or too many calories.

2. The 5:2 diet: Fast for 2 days per week

The 5:2 diet involves typically eating five days a week while reducing calories to 500-600 for two days a week. This diet is also called The Easy Diet and was popularized by Michael Mosley, a British journalist. It is recommended for women to consume 500 calories on the days of fasting and for men to eat 600 calories. You would typically eat every day of the week except Mondays and Thursdays, for example. You eat two small meals for those two days (women's 250 calories per meal and men's 300 calories). No trials are evaluating the 5:2 diet itself, as the detractors correctly point out, but there is plenty of research on the effects of intermittent fasting.

3. Eat-Stop-Eat: Do a 24-hour fast, once or twice a week

Eat-Stop-Eat consists of a 24-hour fast, either once or twice a week. This method was popularized by Brad Pilon, a fitness expert, and has been popular for some years. It leads to a complete 24-hour fast by fasting from dinner one day to dinner the next. When you end dinner, for example, at 7 p.m. Monday and don't have dinner until 7 p.m. the next day, you just did a full24-hour easy. You can fast from breakfast to breakfast, or from lunch to lunch as well. The result is close.During the fast, water, coffee, and other non-caloric drinks are allowed, but no solid foods are allowed.

If you do this to lose weight, you must usually eat during the times of fasting. As in, eat the same amount of food as if you weren't fasting anyway. The potential downside of this approach is that many people may find a complete 24-hour fast relatively challenging.

You don't need to go all - in straight away, though. It's a good beginning with 14-16 hours, and then moving up from there. I have done that a couple of times myself. I found the first part of the fast very easy, but I became ravenously hungry in the last couple of hours.

To complete the full 24 hours, I needed to apply some serious self-discipline, and I often found myself giving up and eating dinner a little earlier.

4. Alternate-day fasting: Fast every other day

Alternate-day fasting means daily fasting. This approach comes in several different versions. Some of them require fasting days to be around 500 calories. Many of the laboratory studies that demonstrated the health benefits of intermittent fasting used some version of this method. Every other day, a complete fast can seem slightly extreme, so it's not recommended for beginners. With this method, several times a week, you'll be going to bed very hungry, which is not very pleasant and probably unsustainable in the long run.

5. The Warrior Diet: Fast during the day, eat a huge meal at night

The Fitness expert Ori Hofmekler popularized the Warrior Diet. During the day, it involves eating small quantities of raw fruits and vegetables and eating one massive meal at night. Basically, within a 4-hour eating window, you "fast" the entire day and "feast" the night. One of the first popular "diets" to include some form of intermittent fasting was the Warrior Diet. This diet also emphasizes food choices that are quite similar to a paleo diet — organic, unprocessed ingredients that mimic what they looked like in the wild.

With some of these approaches, a lot of people get great results. Not everybody gets intermittent fasting. It is not something that anybody has to do. It is just another tool in the toolbox that some people may find useful. Some also think women may not benefit as much as men. This may also not be a safe choice for people who have eating disorders or are susceptible to them.

If you decide to try intermittent fasting, remember to eat healthy too. During the eating periods, it is not possible to binge on junk food and expect to lose weight and improve health. Calories still count, and the quality of food is vital.

Chapter 5:

How To Do Intermittent Fasting For Weight Loss

Fasting is experiencing an increase in popularity, thanks to supporters who say that it promotes weight loss. Everyone seems to be skipping their breakfasts these days or drinking only water every third day. But is fasting healthy for you? And will it (more specifically for some) cause you to lose weight?

The short answer is yes, failure to eat can cause you to lose weight — for a while. Intermittent fasting involves a severe restriction of the intake of food for periods, which induces weight loss. It was primarily a practice associated with religious rituals or other ceremonial activities, until relatively recently. Now it is becoming a lifestyle craze in the mainstream.

If you want to lose fat, then the best strategy is intermittent fasting. Research shows that prolonged fasting — going in and out of the fasting and eating cycles — has enormous benefits for your body and mind. It can ward off chronic illness, enhance memory and brain function, and increase energy levels. What's more, intermittent fasting is an effective way to lose weight and hold it off quickly.

Intermittent fasting will easily monitor your weight loss goals by busting stubborn fat, reducing calories, and re-connecting your metabolism to improve performance. Read on for the theory behind intermittent weight loss and fasting, how to optimize your fast, and a sample routine to get you going.

Intermittent Fasting For Weight Loss

When you're fasting intermittently, you eat all the calories that your body needs but for a shorter period. There are many strategies, but feeding during a 6 to 8-hour period and fasting the remaining 14 to 16 hours is the most common method. It's not as bad as it sounds, especially if you add Coffee to keep the rates of hunger in check (more on that later).

Studies show intermittent fasting speeds up weight loss. The researchers lost a total of 10 pounds in 10 weeks in a 2015 study pooling 40 different studies. One study found that obese adults lose up to 13 pounds over eight weeks after an irregular "alternate day" fasting regimen (consuming 25 percent of their daily calories on one day, and usually eating the next day).

Intermittent fasting also succeeds where many weight-loss regimes fail: by targeting visceral fat and reducing it. Visceral fat is the rigid, tightly compressed inner fat around the abdominal organs. People on an intermittent fasting diet have been able to shed four to seven percent of their visceral fat over six months.

How Does Intermittent Fasting Boost Weight Loss?

Fasting isn't all that unusual if you think about it. Your ancestors had evolved to thrive in rare food situations. Intermittent fasting, in addition to a slew of other health benefits, causes a perfect storm of metabolic changes to combat weight loss and fat reduction. How's it making out?

How To Start Intermittent Fasting

There is no one-size-fits-all when it comes to Intermittent Fasting. Intermittent Fasting suits all your calories into 6 hours, leaving you with a daily 18-hour-fast. This is often termed fasting "18:6." Also, you can try variations like the one-meal-a-day method, or fast every other day — the trick to learning and listening to your body and seeing what works best for you. When intermittent Fasting triggers fatigue or other negative symptoms, try to fast once or twice a week, and then build up from there.

Factors to consider during your fast:

- Prospective Irritability
- Good water consumption

- Ability to differentiate between false hunger and real hunger
- Caloric deficit and resetting of the body's fat-burning hormonal environment.
- Consumption of Amino Acids during "fasting state" (specifically before and after morning "fasted state" workouts.)

Now Let's Look At The Feeding State.

This period for this day will last only the next 6-10 hours, depending on your last meal. It is advisable to consume your three main meals during this time. You still have an aka breakfast (Break the Fast) only later than the usual routine. It doesn't have to include your typical breakfast meal, but if that's your thing, it definitely can.

Every meal is going to be decent in size and will keep you going strong into the next day.

Chapter 6:

What Are The Benefits Of Eating Healthy?

A healthy diet includes a variety of multicolored fruits and vegetables, whole grains and starches, good fats and lean protein. Healthy eating often means avoiding foods, which contain high amounts of salt and sugar. We look at the top 10 advantages of a healthy diet in this review, as well as the facts behind them.

1. Weight loss

Losing weight can help minimize the risk of contracting chronic conditions. If an adult is overweight or obese, they have a higher risk of developing many diseases, including:

- non-insulin-dependent diabetes mellitus
- heart disease
- reduced bone density

Green vegetables and fruits are lower in calories than most processed foods. A person who wants to lose weight should reduce their calorie intake to not more than is needed every day. Determining the calorie requirements of an individual is simple using the dietary guidelines published by the government of the United States. Maintaining a healthy diet free of processed foods will help a person remain under their daily limits without calorie counting.

Fiber is one of the components of a healthy diet, which is especially important for weight management. Plant-based foods contain plenty of dietary fiber, helping to control appetite and making people feel fuller for longer. Researchers found in 2018 that a diet rich in fiber and lean proteins contributed to weight loss without the need for calorie counting.

2. Reduced the risk of cancer

An unhealthy diet habit can lead to obesity, which can increase the risk that a person may develop cancer. Weighing within a healthy range will lower the risk. The American Society of Clinical Oncology has been confirmed in 2014 that obesity was leading to a worse future for people with cancer. All the same, fruit and vegetable-rich diets will help protect against cancer. Researchers have found in a separate 2014 study that a fruit-rich diet reduced the risk of upper gastrointestinal tract cancers. We also observed that a diet rich in vegetables, fruits, and fiber reduced the risk of colorectal cancer and a fiber-rich diet reduced the risk of liver cancer.

Some phytochemicals found in fruits, vegetables, nuts, and legumes act as antioxidants shielding cells from cancer-causing damage. Lycopene and vitamins A, C, and E are some of these antioxidants. Human trials were inconclusive, but the findings of laboratory and animal studies linked certain antioxidants to a reduced incidence of free radical cancer-related damage.

3. Diabetes management

Eating a healthy diet will help a person with diabetes to: reduce weight, if required, maintain blood glucose levels, control blood pressure and put cholesterol levels under target limits to avoid or postpone diabetes complications. It is important for people with diabetes to restrict their consumption of foods with added sugar and salt. Also, fried foods high in saturated and trans fats are best avoided.

4. Heart health and stroke prevention

As many as 92.1 million adults in the U.S. have at least one form of cardiovascular disease according to figures released in 2017. Such disorders affect mainly the arteries of the heart or blood. According to Canada's Heart and Stroke Foundation, up to 80 percent of cases of premature heart disease and stroke can be avoided by making changes in lifestyle, such as through physical activity rates and eating healthily. There are different proof that vitamin E can prevent blood clots, which can result in heart attacks. The following foods contain high vitamin E levels: almond peanuts sunflower seeds. The medical society has long known the link between trans fats and heart-related diseases, such as coronary heart disease.

If a person excludes trans fats from the diet, this will reduce their low-density lipoprotein cholesterol levels. Another form of cholesterol causes plaque to accumulate in the arteries, which raises the risk of heart attack and stroke. Minimize blood pressure can also be essential for cardiac health, and it can help to limit salt intake to 1,500 milligrams daily. Salt is applied to many fried and fast foods and thus should be avoided by a person who wants to reduce their blood pressure.

5. The health of the next generation

Children learn from the adults around them most of the health-related behaviors, and parents who practice healthy eating habits and exercise habits tend to pass these on.

Homemade eating can also help. Researchers found in 2018 that children who often shared meals with their families consumed more greens and less sucrose food than their counterparts who eat less often at home. Additionally, children who participate in home gardening and cooking may be more likely to make healthy choices about their diet and lifestyle.

6. Strong bones and teeth

For strong bones and teeth, a diet with adequate calcium and magnesium is required. It is vital to keep the bones healthy to prevent osteoporosis and osteoarthritis later in life.

The following foods are high in calcium:

- Broccoli
- Cauliflower
- Cabbage
- Canned fish with bones
- Tofu

- Legumes

Besides, calcium fortifies certain cereals and vegetable-based milks.

In many foods, magnesium is available and the best sources are leafy green vegetables, almonds, seeds, and whole grains.

7. Better mood

Emerging evidence suggests that diet and mood are closely related. Researchers found in 2016 that a high-glycemic-loaded diet may cause increased symptoms of depression and fatigue. A high glycemic diet includes numerous refined carbohydrates, such as those found in soft drinks, cakes, white bread, and biscuits. There is a lower glycemic load of vegetables, whole fruit, and whole grains. While a healthy diet can improve general mood, seeking medical care is essential for people with depression.

8. Improved memory

A healthy diet can help prevent cognitive decline and dementia.

A 2015 report identified nutrients and foods that defend themselves against these adverse effects. We considered the following to be beneficial:

- flavonoids and polyphenols
- fish
- vitamin D, C, and E
- omega-3 fatty acids

Among other foods, the Mediterranean diet contains many of these nutritional foods.

9. Gut health Improvement

The colon is made of naturally occurring bacteria, which play significant metabolism and digestion roles. Some bacterial strains also produce vitamins K and B which support the colon. These strains also aid in the fight against bacteria and viruses particles Diet low in fiber and high in fat affects the gut microbiome, resulting in increased inflammation in the area. Diet rich in vegetables, fruits, and grains, however, provides a combination of prebiotics and probiotics that will help good colon bacteria thrive.

Fermented foods are rich in probiotics like yogurt, kimchi, sauerkraut, miso, and kefir. Fiber is a prebiotic that is easily accessible, and rich in legumes, beans, fruits, and green vegetables. Fiber also improves regular bowel movements, which can help prevent diverticulitis and bowel cancer.

10. Getting a good night's sleep

A variety of factors can disturb sleep patterns like sleep apnea. Sleep apnea happens when the airways are crossed again and again during sleep. Risk factors include obesity, alcohol consumption and eating an unhealthy diet. Reducing alcohol and caffeine consumption, whether a person has sleep apnea or not, will help to ensure restful sleep.

Quick tips for a healthful diet

There are many minor, healthy ways to improve the diet, including exchanging soft drinks for water and herbal tea without eating meat for at least 1 day a week, ensuring that intake accounts for approximately 50 percent of each meal swapping cow's milk for plant-based milk eating whole fruits instead of drinking juices that contain less fiber and often include added sugar avoiding processed meats.

A balanced diet can also be given by a doctor or dietitian.

Chapter 7:

Step-By-Step Guide to Intermittent Fasting 16/8

The 16:8 fasting program is a meal regimen in which you fast for 16 hours a day and eat in 8 hours. This diet regimen comes with all the advantages of other fasting schedules (plus, recent research has shown that it will lower blood pressure). Maybe even better, you're going to choose the food slot.

So what's the food window going to be? "There's an endless variety. It can be any day. Any moment you don't eat— that's fasting, fasting specialist, and author of The Complete Guide to Fasting. If you can't live without eating, schedule your meal early in the day (8:00 a.m. to 4:00 p.m.). If you want early dinner, eat in the middle of the day (11:00 a.m. to 6:00 p.m.).

1. Balancing the meals, no snacks between

2. Enrolling 12-12 system

3. BOOM day vol. 1

4. Enrolling 14-10 system

5. BOOM day vol. 2

6. Enrolling into the 16-8.

Balance The Meals, No Snacks Between

So when you decide to start intermittent fasting, test your previous days first. How many meals have you had?

It's all right if you don't know, if you don't remember, or if it all seemed like food all the time. That's the usual situation, as people have hectic lives nowadays.

To continue with, scatter three meals all day and don't have any snacks. Take 3 regular meals, such as breakfast, lunch, and dinner. Don't pay much attention to what you're doing, even if you're meant to get the shakes and carbohydrates out because they're going to make you want to snack and indulge once you start fasting.

Ensure you drink at least 8 cups of water a day. This process should not last more than four days, but if you need more time to adjust, that's great.

Enrolling 12-12 System

After you have learned to have two meals, it is now time to include some laws of intermittent fasting in part. Take three meals and put them in your 12 hours of food slot. And if your first breakfast is 8 a.m., your last meal should not be more than 8 p.m.

You have the sleep time in the 12-hour fasting window.

Make sure you don't eat anything 2 hours before you go to bed! You don't want to sleep after the insulin spike. Let your body accept the food you eat and slowly lower the level of insulin.

This process is estimated to be seven days max.

BOOM Day Vol. 1

Yeah, I made up this name, there's no day like BOOM.

I made that up for a reason. Just when you're happy with the system, BOOM!!! Your body doesn't like booms, even if they're safe like this one.

BOOM Day is simply a fast-extended day.

But you stick to your 12-12 schedule, and it's going to be great. You had your last dinner at 8 p.m. last night. Like you would do it every day, at 8 a.m., you're planning to break the fast. Okay, if you're all right with that, it's time for an upgrade.

Extend your pace for 8 hours.

So instead of splitting it at 8 a.m., break it down at 4 p.m. You're going to get the BOOM part now, don't you?

This isn't going to be easy, so that's what you need. It's easier to have a BOOM day, then to join a complete intermittent fasting schedule at once, and to struggle for weeks. This will cause your body to become frustrated and slip out of the comfort zone. It's going to get to the fat-burning area, and that's when the game starts.

Enrolling 14-10 System

Enrolling the 14-10 program BOOM day is over, and hopefully, you'll be able to break the 20-hour system quickly. You're going to break it now with just 10 hours to destroy the hole.

That's right, no longer than 12 hours to eat. BOOM Day will every the food window by 2 hours, which means that from now on, you're going to fast for 14 hours and eat for 10 hours.

Doing so will help you physically rebound from the BOOM day, so you certainly won't even notice that you're not eating until noon. Note, this is all about loving the process! This time should not last more than seven days.

BOOM Day Vol. 2

Here we're going again. After seven days of the 14-10 system, it's time for another BOOM day, but there's just one tiny little thing I haven't told you yet.

This BOOM day is going to last longer than the previous one. That's why he's had "vol. 2, "but that!

You're going to have to fly for 24 hours.

Surprisingly, this isn't going to be hard, as you might imagine, because you've already conditioned your body to have 0-calories-consuming times. I have fasted more than 24 hours as I did this second day of BOOM. There are two options to do this: PM.

You empty your last meal 2 hours before you leave, you don't eat anything for the whole of the next day, you go to sleep, and when you wake up in the morning, you break the fast.

I will honestly advise you to take option number 2 as the magic happens during sleep time.

As we sleep, our bodies do something like an inventory search. We take all the proteins, sugars, oils, minerals, and vitamins that we got that day, and place them where we belong. Nonetheless, if no food has been processed since the last night of sleep, our bodies will use fat to supply us with energy for the next day. You're losing weight while you're awake.

All choices will show you outcomes, but I do recommend that you take option number two.

Enrolling 16-8 System

And now you're eating intermittently!

Wooooooooooooooooooooo!

Much like the first day of BOOM, you're going to accept these opportunities a lot easier. The principle of intermittent fasting is 16-8, but it can be not very easy to achieve, and this is proved to be the easiest method I've managed to create.

In this process, you're not supposed to eat 3 hours until you sleep, and you should increase your intake of fluids.

You should stick to the 16-8 as much as you want, and even if you choose to update, you don't need to do the BOOM days anymore. Your body has become used to a broader fasting period, so you can gradually increase it.

Talking of an update, there's also an extreme variant of intermittent fasting. It's got a system of 20-4. Indeed, 20 hours of fasting and just 4 hours of food. When you want to do this, get familiar with the 16-8 system first. Push the boundaries for 1 hour if you get relaxed enough with it. You'll be astounded as the pounds fly down!

16:8 Sample Meal Plans.

Right now for the bread. Yes, 16:8 Fasting gives you the freedom to drink what you want while you're sleeping, but it's not an opportunity to go pancake-pizza-Pringles crazy.

"During your feeding times, you need to adhere to a healthy, whole food diet," says functional medicine consultant Will Cole, D.C., IFMCP, "Since some of the effects of fasting include decreased inflammation, piling on junk food during your eating cycle will exacerbate this inflammation. And with inflammation being the underlying factor leading to almost all modern-day health problems, this is something that you want to keep under control. "That means yes to protein purification, healthy fats, so carbs from whole food sources. Skip ultra-processed food and drive-thru; don't skip the emphasis on delicacies. With less time spent on food preparation and planning, it may take a lot of time.

8 a.m.: egg and veggie scramble, side of whole-grain toast

10 a.m.: yogurt and granola

12 p.m.: chicken and veggie stir fry

Evening decaf tea

Midday eating window meal plan

Morning black coffee or tea (no cream or sugar)

11 a.m.: banana peanut butter smoothie

2 p.m.: avocado toast with pistachios

4 p.m.: dark-chocolate-covered almonds

6 p.m.: turkey meatballs and tomato sauce over whole wheat (or zucchini noodle) pasta

Late eating window meal plan

Morning black coffee or tea (no cream or sugar)

1 p.m.: blackberry chia pudding

4 p.m.: black bean quesadilla (cheese of your choice, black beans, bell pepper, and taco seasoning)

6 p.m.: banana

9 p.m.: grilled salmon, vegetables, and quinoa

Chapter 8:
Benefits Of Intermittent Fasting 16/8

IF Helps You Lose Weight Without Following A Traditional, Calorie-Restricted Diet

Research suggests that counting calories and restricting food options will cause stress and increase cortisol levels, which can lead to dietary avoidance, feelings of deprivation, excessive cravings, and regaining weight. Adapting to intermittent fasting, a form of routine eating and fasting depends solely on time. Many people want more flexibility when it comes to losing weight, and they don't want to talk about dieting every day of the week, [because] they lose motivation after a certain period to reduce calories. IF works for people who like to follow the rules, instead of saying' eat less,' we advise them not to eat after 6 p.m., and for those who have the willpower, it really works.

IF Helps You Keep The Weight Off Over The Long Term

On an intermittent-fast diet, it may make it easier to sustain the weight you have gained over the period. A two-part case study of 40 obese adults, published in Frontiers in Physiology in 2016, compared the combined effects of a high-protein, low-calorie, intermittent-fast diet plan with a conventional heart-healthy diet plan. The results showed that while both diets were similarly effective in lowering body mass index (BMI) and blood lipids, those on the IF diet had a benefit in decreasing the loss of weight after one year.

IF May Help Those At Risk For Developing Diabetes

According to the United States of America. The Diseases Control and Prevention (CDC), 84.1 million people in the United States have pre-diabetes, a disease that often leads to type 2 diabetes within five years if not treated. Losing weight, exercising around, and eating a healthy diet will help prevent the development of type 2 diabetes. If you lose weight, you become more sensitive to insulin. It's pushing down the blood sugar.

As we feed, our body releases insulin into the bloodstream to provide the cells with glucose, but those who are pre-diabetes are insulin-resistant, which ensures that their blood sugar levels remain high. Intermittent fasting can benefit those who are pre-diabetic because it allows the body to produce insulin less often. If you are pre-diabetic or have a history of diabetes in your family, this type of diet may be beneficial. Evidence has shown promise in supporting these claims: a study published in the journal Cell in 2017 showed that intermittent fasting cycles could restore insulin secretion and facilitate the law of insulin beta cells in mice with type 1 and type 2 diabetes. While further work is still needed, early studies of human cell samples suggest similar promise.

IF Sync Circadian Rhythm and Shade Away Disease

The internal body clock is a natural system, which regulates sleepiness and wakefulness over a 24-hour cycle. Research published in the 2017 Annual Nutrition Review shows that intermittent fasting can help us adhere to the circadian rhythm of our body and can assist improve our metabolism. Eating these pre-bed foods has also been associated with weight gain and sleep disturbances, mainly when they induce acid reflux. We know that the sensitivity to insulin is improved during the day and that we are less sensitive to insulin at night— the same goes for digestion. This makes you wonder if having dinner at night is going against our body clock. If you want to follow the circadian rhythm, you need to go to bed earlier so that the body can heal itself.

IF May Lower Your Risk For Cardiovascular Disease

According to the CDC, approximately 610,000 people die every year of heart disease in the United States— one in every four deaths. You will reduce the risk of heart disease by adopting a healthy lifestyle: eating right, walking, not smoking, and reducing the intake of alcohol. Research also shows that intermittent fasting can benefit. This increases cardiovascular risk, glycemic control, and insulin resistance if you limit calories every day. In a small study of 32 adults published in the Nutrition Review in 2013, an alternate-day fasting regimen culminated in both weight loss and cardiovascular effects, including increased production of LDL cholesterol and triacylglycerol. Researchers use alternate-day fasting, but keep in mind that fasting doesn't mean not eating — it means eating less. That type of diet is a different way of doing things and may cater to some because they may limit a few days a week rather than every day. As an obese surgeon, I like to have a preference for patients because people are different if it is interesting to you.

Intermittent fasting Increased Growth Hormone

There are very few safe ways to improve your growth hormone levels, so fasting is just one of them. Sufficient levels of Growth Hormone (GH) mean faster regeneration, higher energy, and improved metabolism. The body also uses GH to retain proteins that protect the hair, nails, and skin.

Fortunately, not eating for a long time makes your hormone levels get a real kick. Also, these two studies (here and here) indicate that fasting will increase GH levels by between 300 and 1,205 percent.

Fasting allows you to lose weight, which automatically increases your GH. It also keeps the insulin levels under check so that it does not interfere with the development of GH.

IF May Slow Down The Aging Process

Research shows that intermittent fasting advantages can imitate the results of very-low-calorie diets that are beneficial for anti-aging. A case study published in the Journal of Cell Metabolism in 2014 showed that fasting could slow aging and help prevent and treat disease. It has been shown that fasting causes adaptive cell stress reactions, which result in a better ability to cope with more stimuli and combat disease. "Low-calorie diets improve oxidative stress, and the benefit is anti-aging. The better the mitochondria (the backbone of our cells) work, the better your body works.

IF Works Best For Certain People

Intermittent fasting may offer the greatest benefits to those who are overweight. However, people who have plateaued their weight-loss attempts may notice that intermittent fasting may help jump-start their metabolism and make them grow. It can also help those with digestive problems. Whether you find that your metabolism is late at night, or if you have digestive problems at night, feeding early and fasting overnight might help.

Often attempting a different kind of intermittent fasting is enough for some people to get back on board with their weight-loss goals. One of my nurses gained 30 pounds when she stopped eating late at night. You've got to have that "aah" for a good long-term weight loss."Time, when you remember what was the source of weight gain.

IF Can Reduce Oxidative Stress and Inflammation in The Body

Oxidative stress is one step towards aging and many chronic diseases.

This requires reactive molecules called free radicals, which interfere with and destroy other essential molecules (such as protein and DNA).

Several experiments have shown that intermittent fasting can increase the body's response to oxidative stress.

Some studies have shown that intermittent fasting can help fight inflammation, another key driver of all sorts of common diseases.

IF May be Beneficial For Heart Health

Heart disease is currently the biggest killer in the world.

It is understood that various health indicators (so-called "risk factors") are associated with an increased or decreased risk of heart disease.

Intermittent fasting has been shown to boost several different risk factors, including blood pressure, HDL and LDL cholesterol, blood triglycerides, and blood sugar levels.

Nevertheless, much of this is based on animal experiments. Effects on heart health need to be further investigated in humans before guidelines can be made.

Save A Lot Of Time (And Money)

Eating healthy requires a lot of food preparation that is very time-consuming for many people. I just view Josh Brolin being asked about his Deadpool 2 diet, and he seemed irritated that he had to feed every two hours.

By fasting, though, you save a lot of time and have more fun. Instead of cooking five to six meals a day, you can only cook one or two meals. Not will this only save you time, but you will also love what you eat a lot more as you blend your daily macros in less, but much more abundant, meals.

IF Induces Various Cellular Repair Processes

As we fly, the cells in the body start the cycle of the cell "waste removal" called autophagy.

It includes cells that break down and metabolize damaged and dysfunctional proteins that build up within cells over time.

High rate autophagy may protect against several diseases, including cancer and Alzheimer's.

IF is Good For Your Brain

What is good for the body is often useful for the brain, too.

Intermittent fasting increases the multiple metabolic characteristics considered to be essential for brain health.

It involves decreased oxidative stress, lowered inflammation, and lower blood sugar levels, and insulin resistance.

Several experiments in rats have shown that intermittent fasting may increase the growth of new nerve cells, which are supposed to improve brain function.

It also raises the levels of a brain hormone called a brain-derived neurotrophic factor (BDNF), a dysfunction that has been linked to depression and many other brain problems.

Animal studies have also shown that intermittent fasting protects against stroke injury.

IF Can Improve Your Libido.

I'm going to fully understand if you're a feminist who doesn't want more hormones in her body. But the fact is, both women and men need testosterone in their bodies because of its many advantages, especially for men.

Proper T rates will make you leaner, enhance your bone strength, and improve your libido for men. Men with high T levels typically have a high sex drive compared to men with low T levels who usually suffer from mood swings and, likely, depression. Growth Hormone often comes with a similar increase in T levels. And as intermittent fasting increases GH rates, it means that your T remains at an optimum level.

IF May Help Prevent Alzheimer's Disease

Alzheimer's disease is the most neurodegenerative disease in the world.

There is no treatment available for Alzheimer's, so stopping it from occurring in the first place is essential.

Research in rats showed that intermittent fasting could delay the onset of Alzheimer's disease or reduce its severity.

In a variety of case reports, dietary therapy requiring regular short-term rapids was able to significantly improve Alzheimer's symptoms across 9 out of 10 cases.

Animal studies also indicate that fasting can protect against other neurodegenerative diseases, including Parkinson's and Huntington's.

IF May Cure Fatty Livers

Fatty liver happens as fat is more than 5% to 10% of the weight of your liver. This occurs to heavy drinkers and overweight people when the body is unable to metabolize fat fast enough and, if left untreated, the fatty liver will turn into cirrhosis.

What does fasting sell the fatty liver to you?

According to a 2016 case study by the German Environmental Health Research Centre, fasting helps the liver give a protein called GADD45b (Growth Arrest and DNA Damage-inducible) responsible for regulating the synthesis of fatty acids in the liver. The increase in this GADD45b protein in your body normalizes the fat content of the liver and decreases the amount of sugar in your blood.

IF May Extend Your Lifespan, Helping You Live Longer

One of the most promising aspects of intermittent fasting may be its potential to prolong the lifetime.

Studies in rodents have shown that intermittent fasting increases lifespan in the same manner as constant calorie restriction.

In some of these trials, the results have been quite drastic. In one of them, the rats who fasted every other day lived 83 percent longer than the rats who did not fast.

While this is far from established in humans, intermittent fasting has become very common among the anti-aging crowd.

Given the known effects of metabolism and all sorts of health markers, it makes sense that intermittent fasting will help you live longer and healthier lives.

Chapter 9:
Potential Mistake And Downside Of
Intermittent Fasting 16/8

A lot of people are looking to lose weight. Fasting, voluntary abstention from food, is a common form of weight loss with a long record of success. Nonetheless, many people forget about the cardinal rule of Fasting, or indeed about any dietary change—make sure you do it safely.

But, taken to extremes, Fasting can also have its risks. This is valid not only for Fasting but for anything. When you take veganism to heights, you may be at risk of vitamin B12 deficiency, for example. When you make a low-fat diet to extremes, you are at risk of vitamin D deficiency. When you take the salt limitation to limits, you may be at risk of quantity depletion. When you take extreme activity, you may be at risk for muscle breakdown. must be done responsibly, with knowledge and common sense.

Fasting isn't any different. Since Fasting is already more rigorous than most diets, bringing Fasting to extremes can be troublesome. The film explores some of the risks of Fasting and examines many of the fasting alternatives that are common and may be beneficial to people. Simply put, Fasting is a tool to be used in the fight against obesity-related conditions and perhaps some age-related conditions.

But, like any knife, it's got two sides. It has potential power, and that power can be used constructively, and it can also be used destructively in the wrong hands. It's all a matter of applicability. Most of the resurgence of interest in fasting as a therapeutic alternative revolves on intermittent Fasting—generally shorter duration, regularly and often. The 5:2 diet is two days of Fasting per week, but the fasting days only require 500 calories per day. A time-limited diet, such as a 16:8 regimen, requires you to eat just 8 hours a day so that 16 hours of Fasting is expended. A lot of 24-hour to 36-hour fasts 2-3 days a week, and this is performed under medical supervision with your doctor.

For example, I also use prolonged Fasting, but generally limited to 7-14 days, only in the appropriate person and under observation. Longer speeds have more power, but more risk. To me, there is no reason to run to 30 consecutive days just for the sake of contention. Why not make 4 different 7-day fasts instead? It will have roughly the same positive health effects with a much lower risk.

In Fasting, on the other side, there was a young lady who decided to join a 30-day water-only fasting retreat. As far as I can say, there was no medical monitoring, and there were no blood tests being reviewed, and there was no specialist who even decided whether it was necessary. One of my crucial fasting principles is that if someone is underweight or is worried about malnutrition, they shouldn't be easy. Underweight is characterized by the Body Mass Index < 18.5, but for a safety margin, I do not recommend that anyone be fast more than 24 hours if they have a BMI < 20. The logic seems quite clear. During the fasting period, the body must withstand the accumulation of nutrients and energy. If you have an excess of body fat (stored food energy), then you should be fine. If you don't have a lot of body fat, then it's not all that. It's dumb, man.

Citizens get into trouble with deep rapids because they don't practice common sense. Many of these fasting retreats give only fasts for 30 days of water. If you become sodium-depleted (very common), there are no doctors there to check for warning signs. If you become exhausted and unable to get out of bed, there is something wrong, and you should not carry on Fasting. Okay, that's common sense. With my IDM system, people know that they may feel hungry, maybe a little irritable, constipated, but they shouldn't feel UNWELL. If you really feel bad, you've got to stop. There is no need to go on because Fasting is easy. It's much better to stop and try again (if you want) in a couple of days when you're feeling better. The issue with these fasting retreats is that people have paid money to be there and are therefore going far beyond the boundaries of good safety practice and far beyond the limits of common sense.

Therefore, people practice intense Fasting without any planning. Instead of pursuing shorter speeds and slowly extending them, they quickly opted for a complete water-only extended rate. It's like an inexperienced mountaineer who wants to attempt Mount

Everest, without oxygen and drive it to the summit, whatever the conditions. The seasoned mountaineer will immediately recognize this as a wish to die, but the novice has no inkling of the risks and may come home in a body bag. It's a pure stupid thing. But fasting hospitals are spreading the same notion. Take the most severe fast (water-only Fasting, as opposed to allowing any bone marrow or caloric intake) for an extended period (30 days instead of 1-2 days) in anyone, irrespective of whether this is medically appropriate, without adequate medical monitoring or access to blood work? For now, I can assure you, that's pure stupidity.

Call the marathon story. According to myth, in 490 BC, the Greek hero Pheidippides raced about 26 miles from the frontline near the town of Marathon to Athens to send news of the defeat of the Persians. He roared at Niki! (Victory) and then he knelt instantly and collapsed.

Suppose a sedentary, middle-aged, out-of-shape guy decided to run 26 miles at maximum speed tomorrow, without any kind of planning or awareness. He could keel over and die, too. Nonetheless, in 2014, a 42-year-old man died after the London Marathon, the second death of the race in three years. Earlier that year, a 31-year-old man and a 35-year-old man died in North Carolina. Because the marathon is a relatively extreme occurrence for most people, it takes some planning to be done safely. That's easy to understand, but you can't see the hysteric headlines saying, "Playing, the riskiest thing ever." If you want to hide for a few minutes, you certainly won't be killed. Running a marathon in a new state could do that very well.

The bottom line, though, is that Fasting, done correctly and with knowledge, is an effective factor in the fight against diseases and obesity. Yet devices can cut both ways, and they can sometimes damage the user. A chainsaw is a powerful tool to cut branches. It can also kill you if it is misused. But the right lesson is not to leave the chainsaw. Alternatively, we need to know how to use the tool properly. Fasting used safely, maybe a powerful force for wellbeing. Fasting, misused, will hurt or kill you — fasting by beginning to skip a meal here and there—a good idea. Fasting by beginning 30 days without water is quickly approaching hell or high water—a bad idea.

Chances are, you've come to this book because you're having trouble with your fast — you're not seeing the weight come off, your appetite isn't improving, and you're depressed for most hours of the day.

We're going to dive into the most common intermittent fasting errors you're likely to make and how to correct them.

Intermittent Fasting (IMF) is not a diet, and it is a method of feeding. Most specifically, this is a way of life. It doesn't have anything to partaking with the food you should consume, but when you have this. Relatively simple and straightforward, the 16/8 approach is the most common way to achieve sporadic rpm. It includes skipping breakfast and feeding only in the 8-hour duration of the day while fasting for the other 16.

Since intermittent fasting does not lead to extensive research, it is difficult to provide conclusive evidence. Remember the end goal of improving the body's structure and giving it a standard refresh every day. IF is by no means a one-size-fits-all lifestyle. But it's worth a try!

Overeating

This is one of, if not the most essential, intermittent fasting errors that we see people making as they start implementing the IMF. If you don't consume a healthy amount of food while you're sleeping, that can make you feel thirsty for AF while you're quick, in effect, leading you to overeat right at noon. Have you been going overboard? Chances are you've been sabotaging your rhythm (and your metabolism) along with it.

Overeating is mainly due to our emotional response to fasting. In a world where food is available at our disposal, readily available in our refrigerators, and with a click of a button shipped to our house, we're used to seeing food all the time. If you run, the brain thinks differently, and when you stop eating, it tricks you into believing that you have to eat as much of you as you can in a state of starvation. This is called binging, too.

Say you're used to consuming 2,000 calories a day, and you're starting to fly. You're going for 12-16 hours without eating, you've had your first bite of food at 11 a.m., and the next thing, you've lost your lunch and your best friends, and you can't satisfy that appetite. You're eating so much, you don't want to feed again (like any little meals in the afternoon), and you're eating another big dinner because you're feeling so thirsty when you're out of college. Next thing you know, by the end of the day, you've eaten two huge meals consisting of 3,000 calories and the start of your next easy. You feel like crap, you sleep like garbage, and you can't eat anything for the next 12 hours. See the spiritual environment that you just poured yourself into?

Take it easy on your carbs, pal. My advice is to eat 2-3 medium-sized meals in your fast and have a healthy snack or two in-between. Program your brain, and your body will obey.

Under-eating

Calorie reduction is an efficient way to lose weight, but it can lead to unintended effects when combined with intermittent fasting. It leads to under-eating during your 8-hour period, and if you're under-eating and high, your body can fail, hang on to body fat, and actively try to get rid of muscle. Yes! Yeah! Think about the opposite effect you're going to have, huh?

For short, if you don't eat plenty, you're going to gain weight. Fasting is going against the natural physical cues (like appetite or fullness), so it's essential to understand how much (and what) you need to consume while you're fasting. The best way to do that? Getting a diet consultant, help you out and develop a plan that fits your desires and expectations when it comes to your intermittent fasting and body goals.

Eating too early

You want to deplete as much glycogen as you can all day, so that means you'll move your meal window until later in the day. How can that help you? Okay, let's look at an example of this. Think the fasting time is 4 p.m. It's at 8 a.m. And your breakfast time is 8 a.m. Around four o'clock.

As a general guideline, it takes from 6 and 12 hours for your body to get into a rapid state after you've stopped eating, based on what you've already eaten. So at least your body uses glycogen stores for 4 hours after your last meal. But at the moment, you're unconscious.

You're not running around or working out, so you're not using as much glycogen as you could because your body isn't involved. And after you wake up at 8 a.m. You break your fast and your insulin spikes that stop the process of fat burning.

What I recommend is that you have your last meal just before you go to bed. Let's take a look at another example: the fasting time is from 11 p.m. Up to 3 p.m. And the mealtime is 3 p.m. Around 11 p.m. And you're enjoying your last dinner at 10:30 p.m.

While you're asleep, your body is going into a strong rhythm, and by the time you wake up at 8 a.m. You're more than halfway there already.

So, all day long, you're driving, taking the stairs, working out, and just going about your day, and your body is using glycogen stored in your fat cells. By the time you hit your pace at 3 p.m., You helped burn some of the fat in your body.

The Fast Doesn't Work Without The Feast

Fasting is not a magic pill or magic at all. One of the most significant intermittent fasting errors you could make? Ignoring what you eat for the sake of food.

Yeah, we get it, changing habits is challenging, but if you're not willing to improve what you're eating, including enjoying the processed food single pack burritos from the frozen section instead of some oatmeal or eggs and bacon in the morning, then what? Intermittent fasting is probably not going to work for you, and no other diet is going to work until you are genuinely ready to change from eating processed foods to whole foods.

If you forget what you're drinking, this intermittent fasting error is compounded by some significant drawbacks. We're worried about muscle loss, increased body fat, reduced weight loss, and a serious lack of nutrients. You're fasting now, so why make it harder for your body?

Make sure you choose the most nutrient-dense, nourishing food for the celebration process of your day. It contains beef, balanced carbs, healthy fats, and fruit. The better you do this part, the better you're going to make it through your fast without being too hungry or undernourished.

Drinking The Wrong Thing During The Fast

What do you have to drink during intermittent fasting? Great question, guy! Reports are coming out lately that provide users with more statistical evidence that supports what you can and can not drink, but at this moment, the more comfortable you can handle what you drink, the healthier.

Sources of what you can drink during intermittent fasting include:

- Purified Water or Electrolyte Water
- Baking Soda & Water
- Water &Glauber's Salt
- Herbal Teas
- Black Coffee
- Apple Cider Vinegar
- Fasted Lemon & Cayenne Pepper Water

What are you not supposed to drink during your sporadic fast? As a general rule of thumb, you can stay away from sweetener drinks because they will allow the body to respond to insulin (precisely what we're trying to keep away from in a fasted state).

All in all, try not to drink anything with a caloric benefit or anything that will raise the insulin. Avoid this intermittent fasting error and continue in your fast, longer time to reap more benefits.

Many people will argue that, for example, caffeine or lemon water would kill you quickly. Since there is inconclusive evidence and there are several explanations for fasting, we recommend doing what's best for you and your priorities.

You Aren't Moving Your Body

Listen, I think the war is all right. There are people in the world who enjoy gyms. We enjoy sweat and exercise, that's their stuff. And then there are people in the world like me who need a solid kick in the back to get them out for a 20-minute walk.

The bottom line is that if you don't workout or keep your body healthy, you won't grant yourself the best chance of success in the regimen.

As you exercise, you help your body get faster, and you help it deplete its glycogen stores quicker, because when you workout, the body's primary energy supply is glycogen. This is a great reason why you should do your best to work out before you break down easily and even more if you workout in the morning.

Nonetheless, this is not the only alternative. Working out, in general, is good for your health. Yet working out in a fasted state is perfect for losing fat.

Also, you need to find out if you want to see the weight and lack of fat. When you work out before your body reaches a fasted state, you help your body get further into a fasted state by depleting glycogen.

If you're operating in a fasted state, you're making the body burn the glycogen in your fat cells.

IMF Doesn't Fit Your Lifestyle

If the key doesn't suit, why are you still trying to jam it in the door? Intermittent fasting isn't for everyone, despite all the hype, and if you've tried it, and you've done everything you can to make it a success, and you're still having problems, it's all right to get away from it. When you love food, and it's your favorite meal of the day, because it gives you the strength you need to improve your day, then keep on eating it. If you're an athlete who starts at 5 a.m. and squirts on an empty stomach, then' grab the Tina stuff' and go exercise. When you work the night shift, and fasting gives you a significant energy loss, don't do it.

Often we try so hard to achieve our goals that we risk our overall health. This may include your financial, physical, or emotional health. If the IMF doesn't work for you, or even if it does, the most effective way to make a difference in your wellbeing is by eating whole, healthy, and natural foods.

On the other hand, if you try the IMF and it's hard for you because you're starving and don't get where you want to go as soon, give it more than a week or two. Studies show that it takes 28 days to make a pattern stick, and if you're trying to make IF work for you, skip these typical intermittent fasting errors and give it your best shot.

If you want to lose more weight, improve your appetite, and improve your overall health, intermittent fasting can be an excellent option for you, your goals, and your lifestyle. When you find yourself following all the rules, and you don't like them, so know it's just not for you and move on. Our best recommendation is this: listen to your body and be in touch with what you're trying to tell you, not just what you've read online, what some people have said, or what a company is trying to offer you.

Chapter 10:
Dangers Of Intermittent Fasting 16/8

There's some evidence to back it up. A case study published in the journal Obesity showed that participants eat by 8 a.m. And at 2 p.m. We had smaller appetites and less body fat.

Nevertheless, like any diet, intermittent fasting can lead to extreme eating habits.

In some cases, the adverse side effects of fasting may outweigh any potential benefits.

If you're always worried about what to eat next, it could be a sign of orthorexia.

Dieting, in general, can lead to orthorexia, a condition that includes an obsession with healthy eating. Some of the symptoms of orthorexia show the need to think about your food all the time and stress about your next meal.

One of the overarching signs is when the diet starts to become unyielding. It means changing or canceling social outings because they don't suit the eating habits.

Intermittent fasting can disrupt your sleep, which is critical to health.

There is some preliminary evidence that overnight fasting will enhance sleep by preventing you from waking up in the middle of the night. If people start fast early, their food window often begins to close just before they go to bed. It helps them avoid overnight snacks that can improve the quality of their sleep.

Intermittent fasting can also interrupt the sleep cycle or lead to restless nights. Multiple studies have shown that fasting will reduce the amount of REM sleep that is assumed to improve memory, mood, and cognitive ability.

It could also make you less aware.

Intermittent fasting may contribute to diminished alertness, as the body does not eat enough calories during a fasting period to provide enough strength. Fasting could also lead to exhaustion, difficulties in focusing, or dizziness.

Your diet shouldn't include self-shaming.

If people give themselves a window of time to eat, they will begin to feel bad for breaking their fast too early or eating too late, Rumsey said. Any fear or embarrassment about your diet can be a warning sign of dysfunctional behavior, she said. It involves thinking to yourself when you're waiting for another symptom of orthorexia.

IF can increase levels of cortisol, making you stressed.

Early research has shown that intermittent fasting can reduce the risk of diabetes, obesity, and heart disease, which can lead to increased levels of cortisol, the body's stress hormone, being deprived of food for a more extended period.

Even if there are theoretically any positive health effects, the rise in tension will counteract them.

If you lose your period, it could be related to fasting.

Intermittent fasting can lead to a calorie deficit in some cases, which can lead to hair loss and prolonged or missing hours. Those on an intermittent fasting diet may also feel colder than usual due to low blood sugar levels.

Anxiety and depression could be a tip-off that your diet isn't healthy.

Intermittent fasting leads to disordered feeding when it begins to affect one's health. It involves a difference in mental and social activity, such as a rise in anxiety and depression.

If you feel "hangry," you might want to consider putting a stop.

We've just got a natural night quick while we sleep. Normally, I don't advocate any kind of strict fasting outside of that, because what you're doing is suppressing your body's instincts.

Instead, people should listen to their body's natural cues as to whether they're hungry or finished.

Getting hungry is a real thing to do. Individuals can get irritable.

Avoid Fasting If You Have Higher Caloric

Individuals who are underweight, dealing with weight gain, under 18 years of age, pregnant or breastfeeding should not attempt an intermittent fasting diet because they need sufficient calories daily to develop appropriately.

You should stop fasting entirely if you are at risk of eating disorders. Intermittent fasting has a strong correlation with bulimia nervosa, and, as a result, people who are vulnerable to eating disorders should not undergo fasting-related diets. Risk factors for eating disorders include having someone suffering from an eating disorder, perfectionism, impulsivity, and mood disturbance.

You will most likely feel bloated, overeat, dehydrated, exhausted, and irritable. Intermittent fasting is not for the faintness of your spirit, which means if you are not underweight, you are over 18 years, you are not predisposed to eating disorders, and you are not a pregnant or breastfeeding mother, you will most likely have some unwanted side effects.

You will most likely notice that your stomach crumbles during fasting times, mainly if you are used to frequent grazing throughout the day. To prevent these hunger pains during fasting cycles, avoid looking at, tasting, or even thinking about food that can cause the secretion of gastric acid into your stomach and make you feel thirsty.

Non-fast days are not days when you can splurge on whatever you want, as this can lead to weight gain. Fasting can also lead to a high rate in the stress hormone which can lead to even more food cravings. Keep in mind that over-eating and binge eating are two common side effects of intermittent fasting.

Intermittent fasting is sometimes correlated with dehydration because when you don't sleep, you often fail to drink, so it's important to stay adequately hydrated throughout the day through consuming, on average, three liters of water.

You're more likely to feel exhausted because your body is running on less energy than usual, and because fasting will raise stress levels, it can also interrupt your sleep patterns. It is, therefore, essential to follow a safe, regular sleep schedule and adhere to it so that you can feel refreshed daily.

The same biochemistry that controls mood also influences appetite with food intake affecting the function of neurotransmitters such as dopamine and serotonin, which play a role in anxiety and depression.

This means which deregulating your appetite may do the same to your mood, so you're more likely to feel irritable when you're fasting.

The last piece of advice for people who are involved in an intermittent fasting diet is that the consumption of alcohol is reduced only during feeding times. Do not drink alcohol during or shortly after fasting, and even if you drink during your feeding times, keep in mind that drinking alcohol means that you are displacing the potential for adequate nutrition.

Chapter 11:
Tips And Hack To Success Of Intermittent Fasting 16/8

Intermittent fasting, also shortened to "IF," can be a highly effective means of weight loss. However, contrary to what some people say, it is not a form of hunger or poverty. Speak of intermittent fasting more like time-controlled feeding. It doesn't have to be focused on when you don't feed (like starvation), but instead when you do.

Here are some great tips and tricks that will help you adhere to your intermittent fasting goals. These are strategies that are all easy to implement, produce impressive results, and make the diet plan simpler.

Use the method that works for you

There are three main types of intermittent fasting: fasting for 24 hours, once or twice a week, and daily food on the other days.

Eat all of your calories within 8 hours and fast for the other 16 hours of the day.

Restricted calories 1-2 days a week with healthy food for the remaining five days, typically 500-600 calories on restricted days.

Several variables help you determine which form of intermittent fasting would work best for you. Are you an early bird, huh? Should you work a lot of hours? Are you single or have a partner that will be influenced by your eating habits?

Don't panic if it takes a few attempts to find the program that best suits you. The purpose of the IF is to help you live your best life. It can only do it for you if you hold to the program to make your life better, not more burdensome. It's all right to change the feeding schedule while you're fasting intermittently, the important thing is to find the system that works for you. Experimentation is a good thing!

Stay Hydrated!

Water is a vital part of staying alive, and it's especially important when you're fasting. Drinking water regularly all day will not only save you from getting so thirsty, but it will also keep your organs occupied.

Did you know that many times people make a hunger error for starvation? A little desire that creeps through you, dryness in your throat, and a little touch of irritation? This is hunger more often than you would think. If you can drink cold water or ice water, the cold will refresh you more than lukewarm or room temperature water, and it will give your stomach a little shock that will quench your hunger for longer.

Drink at least 64 oz of water a day. When you work out regularly, you'll need more water. Make sure you drink at least a full glass of water before and after your workout, mainly if you can't or don't like to drink water during your workout.

Buy a bottle of water that can hold at least 16 oz of water. You'll need to refill at least four times a day to get your 64 oz, but sometimes emptying and refilling can be a fun challenge. You can gamify the game by giving yourself time limits to drinking each round, or by giving yourself little incentive when you hit your quota early.

Find your unique cycle

Whenever necessary, avoid eating 2-3 hours before you go to bed, but everything else is up to you. It's normal to continue a quick, 24-hour dinner and breakfast with dinner the next night, but it doesn't have to be that way.

If you're an early morning runner or a gym rat, you could get your exercise, eat breakfast, and then track your start time. And, if you've got a hectic work schedule that's especially crazy on a few days of the week, you could have a quick time around the days you can have lunch.

The same principle applies to limited consumption days or8-hour time restrictions. Do not try to force your identity into a structure that is unpleasant or painful.

Don't Rush Yourself

It always takes time to get used to something different, no matter how excited you are or how much you want it to work for you. That definition may be more accurate to our eating habits than to anything else in our lives.

The way we eat is often rooted in us since we are young. Conscious intermittent fasting is not something that our parents teach most of us. It's a process that we learn as adults, even after the complexities of our eating habits have been cemented.

What does it all mean? Beginning Intermittent Fasting is a massive change for you—physically, spiritually, psychologically. It's all right to take it slow and be flexible. Give yourself a break, please!

It is not expected that new drivers will hop into the vehicle and get straight on the highway. Set realistic goals for yourself and let yourself have a learning curve. That's the only way your experiment of Intermittent Fasting can end up as a safe, balanced eating habit.

Hunger Pains? Create a Diversion.

Sometimes the pain of starvation can be severe during intermittent fasting. They will stop you from work or deter you from doing company. An easy and effective way to fight these hunger pains is to create a diversion for your stomach. (2) Make yourself a cup of hot tea—herbal or caffeine, depending on where you're in your day and what you're up to. Tea has almost no calories in it (as long as you don't pour milk or sugar in it), but it will warm your body and fill your stomach. Caffeinated black or green tea is a great way to give you a little lift and concentrate on it. Herbal tea is going to soothe and calm you as you start to wind your day.

Think ahead to your fast break meal – plan it out.

The best thing you can do for yourself with intermittent fasting, especially at the beginning, is to plan your fast-breaking meal. You're likely to feel very hungry the first few times you stick to quick, healthy, in a way you might not have felt before. Planning your fast-breaking lunch ahead of time will help keep you in control of your appetite.

Traps planning will help you avoid the following:

- **Emotional eating:** You're not going to grab the first enticing junk food you see. Keeping junk food out of your home will help you avoid eating physically, but don't feel like you need to hide indoors! There are fast food places all over the world these days, and the temptations to eat are limitless. Let your meal plan keep you focused on target and light.

- **Overeating:** You're going to be less likely to feed with your head and take extra portions that you don't need. Hunger informs the brain that it has to stock up on food if there is another long wait before food is available again. That reflex is a powerful instinct from when humans had to hunt for food and cook, and no food was assured. Preparing your fast-breaking lunch as thoroughly as possible will prevent you from sinking into an ancient desire to eat as much as possible.

- **Psyching yourself out:** Even when it's time to tick, it can feel like it's forever until your next meal during intermittent fasting. But if you know exactly what you're going to do before your tempo is over, you're going to have a much better target. It's going to give you warmth and relieve your innate insecurity about your appetite. We are often our own worst enemy when it comes to the way we eat. There are a thousand different ways to kill yourself when the tempo comes to an end. Providing a simple, easy-to-achieve meal plan for your quick will give you the support you need to stay on the right track.

Eat Heartily: Give Your Stomach Work

The easiest way to keep the hunger pain away is to give your stomach a lot of work to do. Think of your stomach as an active child. The more exciting and stimulating an experience you can give the kid, the more it's functioning and not looking for something else to do. A precocious child can cause a lot of damage in a short period if left unfulfilled. Say that your stomach is the same way–it's left without food to digest, to keep it occupied, it's going to start pestering you for something to do. The longer your stomach sits, the heavier your appetite is, and the worse the hunger pains become.

Keep away from light, airy foods during your last meal before you start a quick snack. You want to eat foods that have real substance to them. We're not thinking about heavy things like cake and pie (although they're good as mild treats), but rather about nutritious foods that your stomach will need to work to break down.

Consider the following types of food:

- **Leafy vegetables** like spinach, broccoli, chard, and dark lettuces.
- **Potatoes** with the skins on; roasting helps keep the most nutrients in.
- **Grains** like brown rice, wheat pasta, and oatmeal.
- **Soups** that combine many of the ingredients above; but be careful – store-bought soups are often loaded with sodium and processed meat.
- **Fruits** that will give you energy like bananas, apples, grapes, and oranges.

Fasting Doesn't Mean Sitting Around

A lot of people are afraid to go out into the world while they're on the hard. There are endless temptations beyond your house. It could be a challenging idea to go out and meet them while you're fasting.

Yet locking yourself inside is not going to help you in the long run. Not only does it push you to feel lonely and isolated, but it could also make you hate fasting for making you stay inside or unwittingly develop a new bad habit that makes you afraid to eat outside your house.

Go out there and live your life! If it's supposed to be a different part of your life, not to deter you from enjoying it. Select places where the temptations may be less or less tempting to you. Bring friends and help for you.

Eat Foods You Love

This trick is the second most important because it's so important not to forget that you're doing Intermittent Fasting to make you feel better. It's supposed to be a happy and pleasant trip, not an endless method of torture.

Intermittent fasting doesn't tell you what you can and can't eat. This makes you know when to eat and at what pace. Of course, eating healthy and nutritious meals will help you lose weight sooner and more quickly, but that doesn't mean you need to eat healthy foods that you dislike.

Your feeding times will feel much more regular and smoother once you stop fasting with food that you enjoy eating. Not a fruit addict, huh? There's no question! Don't you like to eat meat? Get your protein somewhere else.

Water intake is extremely important.

One of the essential factors in any diet plan is to ensure that your body is well hydrated. By actually drinking a glass of water before each meal, the water can reduce your hunger and make you feel better (so you can stop overeating). Water is going to wash out all the toxins, and the hunger level is going to be much lower.

Listen to Your Body

This is the most critical hack of all— it's your "SELF" hack. React to what the body is telling you to do. It's essential to find and stick to a program, but it's not worth physical or emotional pain.

Intermittent fasting is all about motivating yourself to take control of the way you eat. This ensures that you have full permission to make a shift if it's not going well.

Perhaps one day, 24 hours before you need to eat it, you don't make it completely. When 22 o'clock rolls around and your body begs you to feed–it's all right! Don't beat yourself up, man. Make a healthy choice — slice the cucumber, eat the peach, and have a bowl of oatmeal. Decompress, let go of it, and keep moving.

Intermittent Fasting Frequency

There is no appropriate or incorrect solution to an intermittent fasting schedule— there is only a schedule that works best for you. Keep a close eye on your strength, attitude, and weight loss success, observing how various methods impact you physically and mentally.

Many people practice intermittent fasting on a weekly or bi-weekly basis to make the most of the benefits. Below are a couple of fasting plans that might work for you.

Those who observe intermittent fasting daily will typically have a shorter fasting time and a more extended feeding period. Of starters, if you adopt the 16/8 form of intermittent fasting, you can skip breakfast every day, becoming your first meal of the day.

Weekly Fasts

If you choose a fasting window that lasts 24 hours or longer, it is recommended that you only practice intermittent fasting 1–2 times a week. Fasting is more rational than it could cause muscle loss or other adverse effects.

Bi-Weekly Fasts

If your fast lasts 36 or 48 hours, it's best to take a full week or two weeks off between fasts. Start with a more moderate approach, taking two full weeks off between rapids. When the body is more used to training, you should plan for a more aggressive approach, with just one week off in between.

Skipping Meals

If you're new to intermittent fasting and everyday worries you, missing food is a useful shortcut. If you're eating a big meal, try skipping coffee. If you're busy at noon, skip lunch and have an early dinner.

Although conventional wisdom once cautioned that it would never miss food and mark breakfast as the "most important meal of the day," new research contradicts these views. Skipping food will improve your metabolism, not inhibit it. It seems that skipping breakfast might be just as good as skipping dinner, so take your pick.

If you miss one meal, be careful not to overeat the next. The aim of losing food is to become an intelligent eater — to consume only when you're hungry, not because it's "the time" to enjoy a meal. It's not a reason to gorge on your next sit-down lunch or pursue other types of eating disorders.

Skipping Meals Schedule

If you choose to skip meals instead of keeping to a daily fasting schedule, your eating routine could look different every day of the week. Start by missing a meal when you're not hungry, then try to miss a few meals spaced throughout the week.

- Skip breakfast: Eat only lunch and dinner.
- Skip lunch: Eat breakfast, fast throughout the workday, then eat dinner.
- Skip dinner: Enjoy breakfast and lunch, then do an overnight fast.

Chapter 12:
How To Get Motivated

Motivation is what pushes us to make things happen—but keeping motivated is not always straightforward. Motivation is what moves you towards a mission, gets you up in the morning, and keeps you going through a job that is resolved to achieve when things get tough. Nevertheless, inspiration can be both positive and negative:

- Good motives rely on the good things that will happen as you take action. For starters,' Finishing this task means I'm just a step away from being eligible.'
- Negative motives rely on the negative backlash that will result if you don't take action. For example:' If I don't complete this assignment in the next few hours, I'm going to fail my test.

Both negative and positive motives can be successful in different circumstances. It's much better to do something, though, if you want to do it, rather than because you want to stop a particular outcome if you don't. If you don't have an affirmative action plan, using constructive reinforcement will make you feel powerless and can decrease your motivation.

Regardless matter what you're focused on, there's going to be days when you don't feel like showing up. There's going to be exercises you don't feel like having. There are rumors that you don't feel like publishing. There's going to be tasks that you don't feel like doing. And there will be "bad days" where the energies then feelings are in the gutter. Those changes are part of life, and I have to face those emotional struggles just as much as the next person. Nonetheless, I have also developed a system for coping with these "bad days" for the essential things in my life.

HOW TO GET MOTIVATED ON 3 DAYS INTERMITTENT FASTING 16/8

3 Day Intermittent Fast, Day 0

Last Meal

To toast (Mourn?), I had a beautiful and humongous Sunday night meal with some Toblerone and a drink to enjoy. Then I started my 3 days strong. No more frying, cooking, or eating for 72 hours. It's just juice, tea, lemon, and black coffee.

I went to sleep feeling like a marathoner is about to launch his first run.

3 Day Intermittent Fast, Day 1

Setting Off on a Voyage of Self-Discovery

My first day was kind of like that of an early adventurer searching for the New World. I wasn't entering new territory— I'd done fasts 24 hours before — but this time it was different. I didn't turn back this time. I felt anxious and nervous.

Monday morning began with my regular heavy lifting workout at the gym (and a new personal best!), followed by a lot of online computer work.

Things got strange, then.

Something's Missing

Usually, I should have had a large breakfast early in the afternoon, but this time, nothing. It's all black coffee.

That was worse than not to eat was not to have a daily lunch break for me. Instead of catching up on sports and social media while slurping down a smoothie and some bacon, I just kept working. Who would have thought that fasting could lead to more productivity? Surprise!

My girlfriend Kim, who was supposed to be out until Thursday, shocked me by coming home early. And since I didn't tell her about my 3-day quick strategy, she had brought some fresh salmon for dinner. Wow. Damn.

Surprisingly though, even as I watched and tasted her cook and eat her delicious-looking food with lust, I didn't feel hungry. I was feeling good.

3 Day Intermittent Fast, Day 2

Uncharted Territory

What a strange feeling it is to wake up for the first time in my life after a day of zero calories. I may joke that I felt hollow inside, but I didn't think so. I was feeling great. My sleep-tracking ring even said that my sleep quality was 95%.

Feeling Electric From the beginning of day 2 to the conclusion of my 3-day fast, my mind felt electrical. As if I was high on Adderall, I didn't feel so centered in years.

It, I found out later when I read some books on the biology of fasting, is complete to be expected. My brain was running on better gasoline than it used to, and my whole body benefited from hormone boosts.

I worked in a hyper-focused environment all morning. So, when my eyes began to twitch from staring too much at the phone, I went to the nearby beach to unwind. I've been trying to meditate for 20 minutes, and holy hell! At a certain level, I swear to God that I felt heavy. It's incredible.

The First Poor Experience Like Day 1, I certainly didn't make any personal bests in my Day 2 exercise. I felt like I did the day I tried to work out after I took a bus from Lima to Huaraz in Peru (3000 meters or 10,000 feet).

My body felt good, but it didn't have the stamina it usually did. Between one or two lifts, my energy evaporated, and sometimes I became lightheaded to the point of dizziness.

I was happy I had some exercise, but it was the first negative effect I experienced during my three days.

Unusual Day Again, it was a ride not to have my daily food brakes for lunch and dinner. I missed the ritual more than the food itself. I didn't know what I had to do with myself. It was like a double daylight saving time: usually at 11 p.m. I'm ready for bed, but this time I was prepared by 9 p.m. My brain wasn't going to stop humming, though, so I ended up reading in bed for hours.

Oh yeah, and most critically (and disappointingly): no garbage. No number two at all on Day two of my three days fast.

3 Day Fast, Day 3

What the Hell?

Generally, I wake up at 7:15 a.m. Tomorrow, huh? I was up at 5 a.m. and ready to go. My sleep-tracking ring told me that I had a 90% sleep quality.

I wasn't hungry yet, and my mind was sharp. So did my hearing and my sense of smell, which seemed oddly super-powerful. However, my body felt lethargic.

The strangest thought, though? It's my head.

My mouth was like a warehouse in a business that had just gone bankrupt. It's all spice and stretch, and it's ready to go, but it's bare. My air felt oddly new and flat, and my mouth was tense because of a lack of use. Yes, the night before, I asked myself, "Do I need a brush and floss?"Caving In Do you know how weird your teeth were after you take off your braces? Perhaps your arm leg when the doctor has taken your cast?

That's how my stomach felt heavy the last morning of my three days. It had deflated overnight and felt completely weird to me. In my hand, I couldn't stop touching it. Usually, I can do that stupid trick of poking out my stomach like I'm pregnant, but I can't. It wasn't injured or anything. It just felt a little closer than usual, in the right way.

HOW TO GET MOTIVATED ON 7 DAYS INTERMITTENT FASTING 16/8

I don't follow the plan, and I don't count the calories. I watch what I'm doing, and I'm restricting processed foods. Yet lately, I haven't always made the best food choices. Since I was in the mid-30s, my body seems to be much less accommodating of snack foods. I needed a rebuild.

You've probably heard about intermittent fasting advantages and how the culinary strategy deals with combat infections or removes the weight-loss plateau. Recent studies have found the health benefits of fasting, and I decided to try this out for seven days to see if any of the buzzes are real, from better sleep to slimmer waistline.

Therefore, I switched to the 16/8 form of intermittent fasting: fast for 14 to 16 hours (most of them sleeping), and then restrict my feeding time to 8 to 10 hours. I've spent my meals every four hours of the day and cut out treats, particularly those in front of my bed. I committed to continue my fasting time between 7 and 8 p.m.

Fasting isn't ideal for everyone, and if you have diabetes or other health conditions, you can talk to your doctor before you do anything like this. But you need the motivation to make a healthy lifestyle adjustment, this kind of intermittent fasting may be just what you're looking for.

Getting Started

First of all, I hired my sister to help me to hold me responsible. She has a lot of willpower than I do.

Next, I got ready. I've noticed that menu planning and food preparation are necessary if you want to adhere to a balanced eating plan. I prepared a meal plan for each day over the weekend, shopped and chopped. Each meal required protein, unsaturated fat, and sugar, with plenty of fruit and vegetables. For starters, lunch could be two slices of sprouted grain bread topped with half an avocado, spinach, and two slices of turkey with an apple on the side. Non-caffeinated beverages are recommended for coffee, tea, or low calories. Dinners needed to be simple, fast, and child-friendly for most evenings. We had things like chicken stir-fry, rice bowls, salmon and sweet potatoes, or crock-pot chicken and vegetables.

My Results Are In

I felt great for the first few days. Instead, when my body adapted and remembered that it didn't have as much sugar, I became a little sleepy. But towards the end of the second week, I started to feel better and see progress. Find out the benefits: I'm Not Hangry When I usually have a snack on carbs or a piece of fruit, I'm dying of starvation about two hours later. I feel shaky, and I get a bit excited. Despite the four-hour interval of meals during these two weeks, shakiness has never occurred. I was starving for the next day, but I was just hungry enough to want to eat that huge, full meal.

More extreme responses to hunger, such as jitters, irritability (or hanging), and frustration, are caused by a decrease in blood sugar. It often happens to people with diabetes. But even without diabetes, many of us find that a shift in mood comes to us when it's time to eat. It seems like consuming bigger, nutrient-dense meals helped me to keep my blood sugar steady throughout the day, and I didn't experience those more extreme drops.

Learn to Listen to Hunger Cues. Part of my poor food choices is because I'm feeding out of hunger. Understanding that I set a goal, and a meal plan made me wonder if I was starving because I had a granola bar. Listening to my body's hunger, cues only made me eat when I felt I needed it, or when it was impossible to keep my four-hour schedule. I have made better choices, going for food that gives my body more nutrients and regulates blood sugar like almonds, veggies, and hummus instead of empty calories like chips or crackers.

Body improvements While weight loss was not a primary goal, and I gained nearly two pounds and about half an inch away from my hip. Even a minimal weight loss will help your body better regulate insulin and avoid diabetes. With many family members battling diabetes, I'm looking for ways to reduce my risk.

Must Night This has been a shock. Most of the nights, I toss and turn for a long time before I fall asleep. And in the middle of the night, I still wake up. When I stopped eating after dinner, I fell asleep faster and slept longer than I had in years. Less sleep helps me to concentrate better when functioning, and it's the key to preventing chronic illness.

I love sweets, and when I get thirsty, I crave them more. But, as I packed my plate with food such as avocados and bacon, I found that I didn't want candy as much. My sister found many of the same advantages, and she had more stamina and noticed that it helped to rely on healthy foods.

HOW TO GET MOTIVATED ON 30 DAYS INTERMITTENT FASTING 16/8

I completed a 30-day trial with intermittent fasting, testing the version where one fasts for 16 hours and feeds only for 8 hours every day. I'm going to share in this article what the experience was like.

Of the numerous 30-day trials I did, this was one of the simplest, particularly after the first few days of adjustment. I messed up one day for logistical reasons, eating in a 10.5-hour window that day, but otherwise, it was pretty smooth sailing. I got the food window for a few days within 7 hours. The tightest food period I attempted was about 6 hours.

I've had some prior fasting experience, including 17-day fast water in 2016 and 40-day fast water in 2017, so I've gone for long periods without food since. This didn't take a lot of effort in each event, except for the first few days. The same was true with intermittent fasting, even though I had to keep a watchful eye on the food window every day.

Calibrating the Eating Window

I began this experiment by deciding that I would skip breakfast every day, so my first feeding period was 12–8 pm. It was a good place to start, but in reality, it would be relocated later. As noon rolled around, I'd wrap up whatever research I did first, and then I'd have to prepare something to eat. And when I used this time emotionally, I didn't start eating until 12:30 pm or so.

That was all right, but I didn't like the long stretches of the morning with no sleep, so I didn't need to have dinner too late, because I usually go to bed at 10:30 pm. I got used to skipping breakfast, but I felt like I was doing fine with some food in the morning, mainly when I got up early and practiced.

I tried to move the mealtime to 9 am–5 pm earlier. That was all right, too, but planning with Rachelle to have such an early dinner didn't work well. I didn't feel like I was eating the last meal at 4:30 pm. By the time I was trying this more initial window, I'd already got used to waiting longer for food, and I found it hard to adhere to the previous schedule. My first meal was creeping inevitably later anyway.

Finally, I fell into a routine that I liked, even though I changed it a little. I'd only wait until after 10 am for the first breakfast. By the time I take the first bite of food, it was usually about 10:30 am, which allowed me until 6:30 pm to finish the meal. It was an excellent opportunity, and it didn't feel like waiting so long to get up early. If I was hungry in the morning, I could have eaten soon after 10 am. But if I didn't feel like I was starving, or if I was deeply involved in my morning job, I might not be able to eat until 11 am or later. And, after some training and practicing, instead of worrying about the date, I found it easier to worry about the start time, so I didn't go to the first bite of food sooner than 10 am. Once 10 am rolled along, I could quickly make a game of pushing it back a little — by 15 minutes, 30 minutes, or sometimes an hour or more. The downside of putting it back was that I could have dinner later that day if I wanted to.

The Experience

I can't say that this experiment was too good, but it wasn't too bad either. I've heard a lot of hype about this way of eating, but my experience seems pretty dull compared to some. Many days I feel like I could use something to eat in the morning, but most of the time, those feelings were quickly dismissed. All I had to do was fill my mind with something other than rice. Being wrapped up in a creative project was a game.

When the first meal finally came around every day, I enjoyed it more than average. It felt like breaking a fast, even though it was only 16 hours without food.

I always became more conscious of what I was eating, particularly for the first meal of every day. When I was eating at 10:30 a.m., I'd worry about whether I needed to call it breakfast and have some steel-cut oats with fresh berries and coconut milk or call it lunch and have air-cooked tofu or tempeh salad.

Since this encounter disrupted my former food schedule, it made me think about when to eat and pay more attention to how hungry I was, instead of just feeding because it was the regular mealtime.

Mentally, I did not notice any meaningful improvement by eating this way— no improvements of mental clarity that I can detect, but no deterioration either. Nonetheless, by not having an early meal, I save time on food preparation and cooking, so I was able to get going on my working day faster than I needed to.

Weight Loss

Over the last 30 days, I lost a little bit of weight, just 1.6 pounds. But that's only been the last ten days. For the first three weeks, I've been close to my starting weight all the time. Even so, if that weight loss pace were to be maintained for a whole year, it would be 19 pounds, which is not bad for a reasonably easy-to-maintain strategy.

Eating in 8 hours didn't seem particularly advantageous if I just consumed the same amount of food I would have eaten before. It was shockingly easy to eat the same amount of food for the first few weeks. But then I slowly found that I was eating less food than I had before. And that's when I began to see the nudging of my weight. In the long run, though, I think that this type of intermittent fasting will make it easier to lose weight because you're likely to eat fewer calories this way. After a while, it started to feel more effortful to try packing the same amount of food in 8 hours.

I think the key here was to indulge in this way of eating and not to regulate it. Initially, I was dwelling on those 8 hours, and I was worried about when I was supposed to eat my meals during that time as if I had to pre-decide when to feed. Then, I just focused on getting past 10 a.m. and letting my hunger decide when to feed, and that's when this process got better, and I started to lose a little weight.

Sometimes I didn't seem as thirsty as I was before. I ate a banana with some peanut butter for dinner one night, so I didn't want more than that. Some days, I found that I was going for more extended periods without feeding. I might feel empty inside, but I wasn't starving on my own.

Final Thoughts

For the first 20 days, this experiment was almost pointless. I couldn't see any results, and I was still calibrating to find the right food window for me. It was only in the last ten days that I began to notice a few changes. Since then, I had lined up with a meal period that fit perfectly (about 10:30 a.m. to 6:30 p.m.), and I was left with a simple rule: wait until after 10 a.m. before I had some food.

Overall, I believe that 30 days was too little time to draw any conclusions as to what the long-term effects of this way of eating might be. The findings were modest relative to other food studies I've done over the years. The transitions from dairy to organic were much stronger and more visible (like losing 7 pounds in the first week when my body finally lost years of milk clogging).

Nevertheless, this encounter made me curious about intermittent fasting, so I'm likely to continue playing with it. Several people suggested that the food window should be shortened even more, say 4 hours or less. And there are several other combinations to use as well.

I like consistency, so I don't plan to be as rigid about intermittent fasting while driving or on a busy schedule, but the ease of not eating before 10 a.m. has worked pretty well, and it seems pretty easy to keep going.

Chapter 13:
How To Choose Foods

Eating during intermittent fasting (IF) may be frustrating. This is because intermittent fasting is not a diet plan, but a method of feeding. Keeping this in mind, DoFasting experts have developed an intermittent fasting food list that will keep you healthy while you're on your weight loss journey.

Intermittent fasting teaches you when to eat, but it doesn't tell you what foods can be included in your diet. Lack of clear dietary guidelines can give a false impression that you can eat whatever you want. Others may find it challenging to choose "appropriate" foods and drinks.

Not only do they hinder your weight-loss plans, but they can also make you more likely to be undernourished or overnourished.

Eat Real Food

It doesn't take a genius to figure this out. Ultimately, man is never going to improve on what God has made.

"Consume a range of nutrient-dense foods and beverages within and across basic food groups while selecting products that restrict the consumption of saturated and trans fats, cholesterol, added sugars, salt, and alcohol." The dilemma is that common sense must contend with a strong trillion-dollar food industry that is bombarding us with advertisements that are designed to make us consume more and more of the worse things. There is an inverse relationship between nutritional value and income when it comes to food. The more you refine some products, the more you make it profitable. The more it is stored, the less nutritional value it holds. That's why we see stuff like enriched flour. They're trying to put some of the minerals back in that they've been stored. Everything we end up with is a far cry from what God has given us. Packaged and processed food firms waste little effort to push more of their goods into their target market. More than 90% of their merchandise sales are made to less than 10% of their consumers. "In the case of processed food, the desirable 10% consists primarily of people weighing more than 200 pounds and making less than $35,000 per year." No cost is spared to strike any strategic button that matters to the target market. Like a deer captured close to the range of a hunter, the target never has a chance.

Many times, the unhappiness of the cycle threatens the consciences of the $200,000-per-year marketing executives in charge of it. Others also refuse to participate in their focus groups. Instead of addressing their future victims in person, they choose to study documents in the privacy of their workplaces.

One of the major scandals in junk food society is the degree to which its most dedicated advocates ignore the very items they are promoting.

Such food companies are doing something even worse than exploiting low-income, obese, overweight customers for their goods. Once the target enjoys the drug and becomes a consumer, the business chemists guarantee that they will never be content by consuming just a healthy amount of it.

They] have been updated to ensure that "no one can eat just one of them." Such chemical modification induces a great deal of overconsumption, encourages malnutrition, and kills the natural tendency of our taste buds to search for variation in what we consume.

Maybe at this point, you're starting to feel some righteous indignation. We permitted ourselves to be led astray like pigs to the slaughter. I am told again of the words of Jesus, "The robber comes only to steal, and to kill, and to destroy, and I came that they might have life, and have it abundantly" (John 10:10). Such issues aren't meant to shock us. It's our responsibility to educate ourselves so that we learn right from the bad. That takes me back to that point. The only best thing you can do to ensure proper nutrition is to eat predominantly unprocessed whole foods. Real food, non-edible food-like compounds.

If most of your diet consists of real food, you'll get better nutrition and be more comfortable while eating fewer calories. A safe way to make sure you're eating real food is to walk around the store and keep out of the center.

Eating during intermittent fasting is more about being balanced than just dropping your weight quickly. It is, therefore, vitally important to choose nutrient-dense foods such as vegetables, meat, lean proteins, and healthy fats.

The list of intermittent fasting foods will contain:

FOR PROTEIN

The minimum dietary allowance (RDA) for protein is 0.8 grams of protein per kilogram body weight. Your criteria that vary depending on your fitness goals and your level of activity.

Protein helps you lose weight by raising your energy intake, increasing your satiety, and improving your metabolism.

Also, when combined with strength training, improved protein intake helps build muscle. Getting more muscle in your body improves your metabolism because muscle consumes more calories than fat.

A recent study shows that having more muscle in your legs will help reduce the production of stomach fat in healthy men.

The intermittent fasting diet nutrition list includes:

- Poultry and fish
- Eggs
- Seafood
- Dairy products such as milk, yogurt, and cheese
- Seeds and nuts
- Beans and legumes
- Soy
- Whole grains

FOR CARBS

According to the American Dietary Guidelines, 45 to 65 percent of your daily calories will come from carbohydrates (carbs).

Carbs are the primary source of energy for your body. The other two of them are protein and fat. Carbs come in a variety of ways. Sugar, fiber, and starch are the most popular of them.

Carbs often get a bad rap because it causes weight gain. Not all carbs are created equal, however, and they are not necessarily fattening. Whether or not you gain weight depends on the type and quantity of carbohydrates you consume.

Make sure you pick foods that are high in fiber and starch but low in sugar.

A 2015 study suggests that consuming 30 grams of fiber per day can cause weight loss, increase glucose levels, and lower blood pressure.

Getting 30 grams of fiber out of your diet is not an uphill struggle. You will get them by consuming a basic egg sandwich, Moroccan chicory rice, peanut butter pie, and chicken and black peas enchiladas.

The list of intermittent fasting foods for carbs includes:

- Sweet potatoes
- Beetroots
- Quinoa
- Oats
- Brown rice
- Bananas
- Mangoes
- Apples
- Berries
- Kidney beans
- Pears

- Avocado

- Carrots

- Broccoli

- Brussels sprouts

- Almonds

- Chia seeds

- Chickpeas.

FOR FATS

According to the 2015-2020 Dietary Guidelines for Americans, fats are expected to contribute 20% to 35% of your daily calories. Saturated fat should not add more than 10% of calories per day.

Fats can be good, evil, or just in-between depending on the type.

For example, trans fats increase inflammation, reduce "healthy" cholesterol levels, and increase "poor" cholesterol levels. We are used in fried food and baked goods.

Saturated fats can increase the risk of heart disease. Nonetheless, there are varying expert views on this. It's a good idea to eat them in moderation. Red meat, whole milk, coconut oil, and baked goods contain high levels of saturated fat.

Healthy fats are monounsaturated and polyunsaturated fats. Such fats can reduce the risk of heart disease, lower blood pressure, and lower-fat blood levels.

Olive oil, peanut oil, canola oil, safflower oil, sunflower oil, and soya oil are rich sources of these fats.

The list of moderate fasting foods for fats includes:

- Avocados

- Nuts

- Cheese

- Whole eggs

- Dark chocolate
- Fatty fish
- Chia seeds
- Extra virgin olive oil (EVOO)
- Full-fat yogurt.

FOR A HEALTHY GUT

A growing body of evidence shows that your digestive health is the secret to your overall health. The stomach is home to billions of bacteria known as the microbiota.

Such bacteria affect your intestines, your metabolism, and your mental health. These may also have a vital role to play in many psychiatric illnesses.

You can take care of those tiny bugs in your stomach, particularly when you're fasting intermittently.

The list of intermittent fasting foods for healthy intestines includes:
- All vegetables
- Fermented vegetables
- Kefir
- Kimchi
- Kombucha
- Miso
- Sauerkraut
- Tempeh

In addition to keeping your gut healthy, these foods can also help you lose weight by:
- Decreasing the absorption of fat from the gut.
- Increasing the excretion of ingested fat through stools.
- Reducing food intake.

FOR HYDRATION

According to the National Academies of Sciences, Engineering, and Medic͎
fluid requirement is:

- About 15.5 cups (3.7 liters) for men.
- About 11.5 cups (2.7 liters) for women.

Fluids provide liquids as well as food and drinks containing water.

Staying hydrated during intermittent fasting is essential to your wellbeing. Dehydration can cause headaches, extreme tiredness, and dizziness. If you're already dealing with these side effects of fasting, dehydration will make them worse or even more severe.

The intermittent fasting food list for hydration include:

- Water
- Sparkling water
- Black coffee or tea
- Watermelon
- Strawberries
- Cantaloupe
- Peaches
- Oranges
- Skim milk
- Lettuce
- Cucumber
- Celery
- Tomatoes
- Plain yogurt.

Ironically, drinking a lot of water can also help with weight loss. A 2016 review study shows that proper hydration will help you lose weight by:

- Decreasing appetite or food intake.
- Increasing fat burning.

Foods To Exclude From The Intermittent Fasting Food List

- Processed foods
- Refined grains
- Trans-fat
- Sugar-sweetened beverages
- Candy bars
- Processed meat
- Alcoholic beverages.

Combining Intermittent Fasting with Specific Diets: Things to Know

Many people believe that mixing IF with other diets, such as keto diets or vegetarian diets, is more effective in weight loss. That said, the jury is still out on whether this is valid or not.

Do you want to try the mixture of IF and keto diet? Make sure you include the following in the high-fat low-carb diet with intermittent fasting foods:

FOR FATS (75% OF YOUR DAILY CALORIES)

- Avocados
- Nuts
- Cheese
- Whole eggs
- Dark chocolate
- Fatty fish
- Chia seeds
- Extra virgin olive oil (EVOO)
- Full-fat yogurt

FOR PROTEIN (20% OF YOUR DAILY CALORIES)

- Poultry and fish
- Eggs
- Seafood
- Dairy products such as milk, yogurt, and cheese
- Seeds and nuts
- Beans and legumes
- Soy
- Whole grains

FOR CARBS (5% OF YOUR DAILY CALORIES)

- Sweet potatoes
- Beetroots
- Quinoa
- Oats
- Brown rice

The food list for intermittent fasting vegetarian diet includes:

FOR PROTEIN

- Dairy products such as milk, yogurt, and cheese
- Seeds and nuts
- Beans and legumes
- Soy
- Whole grains

FOR CARBS

- Sweet potatoes
- Beetroots

- Quinoa
- Oats
- Brown rice
- Bananas
- Mangoes
- Apples
- Berries
- Kidney beans
- Pears
- Avocado
- Carrots
- Broccoli
- Brussels sprouts
- Almonds
- Chia seeds
- Chickpeas

FOR FATS

- Avocados
- Nuts
- Cheese
- Dark chocolate
- Chia seeds
- Extra virgin olive oil (EVOO)
- Full-fat yogurt.

What To Drink During Intermittent Fasting

Beverages can be a lifesaver when it comes to fighting hunger pangs and cravings in your fasting hours. Some drinks can help improve the results of your intermittent fasting strategy. Nice, nice!

Here are the drinks you can enjoy in your fasting windows:

Water

You will (and should!) drink water during your fasting periods. Water is always a great choice, all day long. It could be still or dazzling, no matter what you like. You can also add a lemon (or lime) squeeze to your drink if you want lemon water. Consider infusing a pitcher of water with cucumber or orange slices for other exciting taste combinations.

Yet make sure you stay away from any artificially-sweetened water enhancers (such as Crystal Light). The artificial sweetener will interfere with your rhythm!

Coffee

Black coffee is a calorie-free product that does not affect insulin levels. During the fasting hours, you should drink regular coffee (caffeinated) or decaf coffee, don't add any sweetener or sugar. Spices like cinnamon are all that!

Most coffee drinkers enjoy a cup of joe, or even espresso, in fasting periods with no adverse effects. But some people have a pounding pulse or an upset stomach as they drink coffee in fasting hours, so watch your own experience.

Bonus: Black coffee may enhance some of the benefits of intermittent fasting, and it's quite popular with people who also adopt a keto diet. This research has shown that taking caffeine will help with the development of ketone. Coffee has also been shown to improve long-term stable blood sugar levels.

Bone Broth

Bone broth (or vegetable broth) is recommended at any time you decide to fast for 24 hours or more.

Beware of frozen broths or blocks of broth! These have lots of artificial flavors and preservatives that will counteract the effects of your speed. A good homemade soup, or a foundation of confidence, is the way to go.

Tea

Help increase your satiety with tea, of course! It could just be the secret weapon that makes the fasting strategy simpler but also more effective.

All kinds of tea are perfect for a quick drink, like white, black, oolong, and herbal teas. Tea increases the efficacy of intermittent fasting by encouraging digestive health, probiotic balance, and cellular safety.

Green tea, in particular, has been shown to help increase satiety and promote healthy weight management.

Apple Cider Vinegar

Drinking apple cider vinegar has several health advantages, and you can continue drinking it while fasting intermittently, even during fasting periods. And since ACV helps promote healthy blood sugar and digestion, it may also improve the benefits of your intermittent fasting strategy.

If you're not a fan of apple cider vinegar, use it as a salad dressing while you're chewing glass. It's perfect for you at every time of the day.

Are there any drinks that you should stop during intermittent fasting?

There are a few drinks (including "zero-calories") that you may not know are capable of "breaking the fast." That means that if you eat them, you're going to get your body out of the "hot zone."

Chapter 14:
Importance Of Healthy Lifestyle

Living is all about consensus. Okay, if you believe that you can ignore your bad eating habits just because you exercise regularly, think again. A mistake more people make is to believe that if you lose a lot of calories in the gym, you can eat whatever you want. And, if you're "naturally" thin, you don't have to watch what you're doing. Sadly, trading an hour in the gym for a greasy double cheeseburger or depending on a high diet to take the place of healthy eating habits completely misses the point of living a healthy lifestyle the most important thing you can do is to eat well. Evite contaminants in your diet as much as possible and drink plenty of fresh fruit, vegetables, and whole grains; exercise regularly a few days a week; avoid smoking, even second-hand smoke; and avoid adding too much weight (which should come naturally if you eat well and exercise). While it is not necessarily possible to eat all organic food-the EEC suggests 12 organic fruits and vegetables because of their higher levels of pesticide residues.

Our modern lifestyle is very convenient, but it can also be very unhealthful. Most people eat too many processed foods and too few fruit and vegetables; we never exercise, and when we encounter chronic conditions such as diabetes, we rely on prescription drugs to make us feel better-but these medications often have harmful side effects. Instead of acknowledging the value of living a healthy lifestyle for us and future generations, we perpetuate our bad habits-and then taking potent, dangerous drugs to treat our last symptoms.

Of example, not all facets of a healthy lifestyle are in our power. We will be exposed to certain environmental toxins, whether we like them or not. But many of these variables are totally beyond our influence. Whenever we can, we need to be cautious and make the right choices.

That's why it's so important to be sure that you're eating well as a critical factor in keeping a healthy lifestyle.

Eating a healthy diet is far from essential, simply because people are very complex beings. They may have it in the back of our minds that they consume to sustain our bodies, but we make the majority of our food choices based on their pleasure aspect. Eating is such a pleasant experience that we often choose to eat food that tastes very nice, but that doesn't make us feel very well afterward. They also love these things so much that they eat more than our bodies require, which leaves us overweight, sad, and stressed.

You know that a healthy lifestyle, such as eating right, exercising, and eliminating harmful substances, makes sense, but have you ever stopped thinking about why you pursue them? Every activity that supports your physical, behavioral, and emotional health is a healthy habit. Those activities should enhance your general well-being and make you feel good.

Healthy lifestyles are challenging to develop and often require a change of mind. However, if you're willing to make sacrifices to improve your health, the effect can be far-reaching, regardless of age, race, or physical ability. Here is the value of a healthy lifestyle.

Controls weight

Eating right and exercising regularly will help you avoid excess weight gain and maintain healthy body weight. Getting physically active is key to meeting your weight-loss aim. Even if you're not trying to lose weight, regular exercise will enhance your cardiovascular health, strengthen your immune system, and increase your stamina.

Prepare for at least 150 minutes of moderate physical activity each week. When you can't dedicate this amount of time to fitness, search for an easy way to increase movement throughout the day. For starters, try walking instead of driving, take the stairs instead of the elevator, or pacing while you're talking on the phone.

Eating a healthy calorie-driven diet can also help control weight. If you start your day with a healthy breakfast, you stop being too hungry later, which might send you off to get fast food before lunch.

Skipping breakfast will increase blood sugar, which decreases fat storage. Such foods, which are low in calories and rich in nutrients, help to control weight. Reduce the use of sugary drinks, such as sodas and fruit juices, and choose lean meats such as tuna and turkey.

Improves mood

Doing right with your body pays off for your mind as well. The Mayo Clinic states that physical activity increases the development of endorphins. Endorphins are brain chemicals that make you feel better and more comfortable. Eating a healthy diet as well as exercise will lead to a better body. You're going to feel better about your looks, which can improve your confidence and self-esteem. The short-term benefits of exercise include decreased depression and increased cognitive function.

It's not just diet and exercise that leads to a better attitude. Social connections are another healthy habit that leads to better mental health. Either volunteering, joining a club, or taking part in a film, social tasks help to improve morale and mental functioning by keeping the mind active and the amount of serotonin controlled. Don't just remove yourself. Spend time with your family or friends regularly; if not every day. If there is a physical barrier between you and your loved ones, using apps to stay connected. Pick up your phone or start a video chat.

Combats diseases

Healthy habits help prevent such aspects of health, such as heart disease, stroke, and high blood pressure. You will keep your cholesterol and blood pressure within a safe range if you take care of yourself. It keeps your blood flowing steadily, reducing the risk of cardiovascular disease.

Regular physical activity and a proper diet can also avoid or allow you to control a wide range of health issues, including:

Metabolic syndrome

Diabetes

Depression

Certain types of cancer

Arthritis

Make sure that you book a physical exam every year. The doctor will monitor the weight, pulse, and blood pressure, and take a sample of your urine and blood.

Boosts energy

Since overeating unsafe food, we've all felt a lethargic sensation. If you eat a balanced diet, your body gets the fuel it needs to control its energy level. A healthy diet includes the following:

Whole grains

Lean meats

Low-fat dairy products

Fruit

Vegetables.

Regular physical training also increases muscle strength and endurance, giving you more capacity, says Mayo Clinic. Exercise helps bring oxygen and nutrients to your tissues and gets your cardiovascular system to work more efficiently so that you have more time to do your daily work. It also helps to boost efficiency by encouraging better sleep. It allows you to fall asleep quicker and get a deeper sleep.

Insufficient sleep can give rise to a variety of problems. Apart from feeling tired and sluggish, if you don't get enough sleep, you may also feel irritable and moody. Also, poor sleep quality may be responsible for high blood pressure, diabetes, and heart disease and may even shorten your life expectancy. To improve the quality of sleep, adhere to the routine where you wake up and go to bed at the same time every night. Reduce the intake of caffeine, restrict the napping, and build a comfortable sleeping atmosphere. Turn off the lights and the Radio, and keep the room temperature high.

Improves longevity

Once you adopt healthy habits, you increase your chances of a longer life. The American Exercise Council conducted an 8-year survey involving 13,000 men. The study showed that those who exercised just 30 minutes a day significantly reduced their chances of dying prematurely compared to those who practiced occasionally.

Looking forward to more time with your loved ones is reason enough to keep going. Start with quick5-minute walks and gradually increase the time to 30 minutes.

Strive For A Healthy Lifestyle

It's commitment and not always enjoyable, so why worry? At some point in your life, you will face the revelation that your body's health is the determining factor in what kind of lifestyle you will live. Just as a smoker faces a possible future of emphysema and lung cancer, if you lack healthy eating habits, not only do you face a possible future of overweight or obese, you always run the risk of insomnia, heart disease, diabetes, stroke, digestive problems and more. The choices you make every day—from what to eat for breakfast and whether or not to have an extra slice of pie—affect how you feel and how you act, which, as you may be able to guess, changes everything you do. Choose carefully, and eventually, you will realize that feeding your body well turns into a better, safer, more enjoyable life.

When you agree that learning healthy eating habits is worth it to you, it's time to make some adjustments to your eating. Dare yourself to come up with some new healthy eating habits every day and put them to good use, including drinking more water or using mustard instead of mayonnaise on your sandwiches. Rather than trying to cut out all the "bad" things you're currently eating, such as many processed foods, cookies, soda, candy, and other junk foods, it's much more comfortable and safer to start putting more healthy meals, such as fresh fruits and green vegetables, whole grains, lean meats, low-fat dairy products, nuts, and legumes. This way, you're slowly replacing your bad diet with a proper diet, and you're not left with a big, gaping void where your bad food was once. Once you start filling in healthier foods, it's harder for you to let go of some of the more common dangerous foods.

Tips for Beginning a Healthy Lifestyle

1. Prepare the routine of workouts. Prepare your weekly schedule just like you do with college. Consider your safety and yourself a priority. Schedule training sessions daily just as you would have a fitness group. Commit to your exercises.

2. Get a mate of your exercise. Family and mates are a great place to get going. Getting a fitness partner will help motivate you, drive you, and lead you through workouts. Working with someone else helps to keep you accountable. You're more likely to stay on board when someone else is counting on you for an exercise.

3. Find a class that will inspire you. What kind of exercise is going to get you to the gym? The most important thing at the outset and throughout your healthy lifestyle is to engage in activities and events that inspire you to walk around. Would you enjoy aerobic dance classes, body sculpting courses, or a boot camp at the local gym? Determine the thing that

you would like to do the most and gravitate to that task. Sessions are a perfect way to get started. Classes provide a coach to help motivate you to keep your exercises healthy to avoid injury.

4. Get active in a group or game. Have you dreamed of getting involved in activities like basketball, pool, baseball, softball, or running a club? Organized sports events and clubs provide an excellent environment for engaging with like-minded people. Sporting organizations and activities are the best way to keep you involved, motivated, and on a training schedule.

5. Set short-term and long-term goals. First and foremost, it's essential to be realistic about your goals. If your goals are to lose weight, boost fitness, compete in athletics, or just become more social, goals can be a great way to keep you on track. Make sure you monitor your success as well. Whether you're checking on your milestones or making a diary or using an app on your phone, keep track of the actions you're doing to achieve your goals and by what date you'd like to achieve your goals. That person is different, and the expectations of each person should be unique to you and your health and lifestyle.

6. Adopting healthy eating habits. Not only are the workouts important, but healthy eating is also essential. If you want to boost your fitness, lose weight, and become safer, you'll need to fuel your body properly. Make sure you hydrate, eat whole fresh foods and try to remove processed foods from your diet. Prepare your weekly menus, log your diet every day, and note to thank you for all your hard work at the end of each week. Note, it's about lifestyle, not poverty.

A healthy lifestyle is not going to happen overnight. But with a regular exercise schedule, healthy eating, and healthy eating habits, you're one step closer to your target. Sit down and work out a workout schedule and a healthy eating schedule. Getting organized will help you stay on track and make sure you stick to your new healthy routine.

Healthy Lifestyle Make Differences

Okay, as it turned out, a healthy lifestyle makes a big difference. According to this study, people who met requirements for all lifestyles lived substantially, impressively longer lives than those who did not have: 14 years for women and 12 years for men (if they had this lifestyle at the age of 50). People who did not have any of these patterns were much more likely to die early from cancer or cardiovascular disease.

The authors also measured life expectancy from how many of these five healthy habits people have. Just one healthy lifestyle (and it doesn't matter which one) only one extended life expectancy of men and women by two years. Not unexpectedly, the healthier lifestyle people have longer their lives.

Okay, this is massive. However, it supports earlier, similar research— a ton of earlier, related research. A 2017 study using data from the Health and Retirement Study found that people 50 and older, who were of normal weight, had never drunk and had regularly drunk alcohol, lived an average of seven years longer. A 2012 mega-analysis of 15 international studies comprising more than 500,000 people showed that more than half of early deaths were due to unhealthful lifestyle factors such as poor diet, inactivity, obesity, excessive alcohol consumption, and smoking. And the list of research aids continues.

Chapter 15:
Importance Of Regular Weight

When you grow older, if you continue to eat the same kinds and amounts of food but do not become more involved, you are likely to gain weight. That's because your metabolism will slow down with age, and body composition may be different from when you were younger.

The nutrition that the body derives from the nutrients in the meals you consume is known as calories. As a rule of thumb, the more calories you consume, the more healthy you have to keep your weight. Likewise, the reverse is true— the more involved you are, the more calories you use. The bodies may need less food for energy when you mature, but it still needs the same amount of nutrients.

Decreased Breast Cancer Risk

Overweight can increase the chances of breast cancer by 30 to 50 percent, according to the Cancer Prevention Organization.

Improved Heart Health

A record published in the Journal of the American College of Cardiology, which looked at almost 15,000 relatively stable Korean individuals with no documented heart disease, shows that those with the body mass index (BMI) of more than 30 were more likely to show signs of early plate build-up in their arteries than normal-weight people. This has prompted researchers to believe that, although these individuals may have been metabolically stable at the time of the test, their weight is likely to have negative consequences on their health still.

More Motivation

A study of Obesity shows that overweight women's brains respond negatively to the idea of working out— but that people's photos favorably influence women's brains that are at a healthy weight in the middle of a workout session.

Increased Fertility

The ideal weight — in terms of pregnancy — is the BMI between 20 and 24, say, fertility experts. The American Society for Reproductive Medicine currently reports that 12% of cases of infertility are due to weight-related problems (about the same number of people who have infertility are overweight and underweight). Why? Why? Your weight will affect your cycles and ovulation— so if you don't have a regular beating, your fertility can fail.

Better Sleep

According to a 2012 study, weight loss— particularly nasty abdominal fat — may help you record higher-quality fat. Fat, and specifically belly weight, interferes with lung function, making it harder for the lungs to expand because fat is in the way. And since breathing problems can lead to nighttime complications such as sleep apnea, it takes a toll on your eyesight.

Decreased Risk of Diabetes

In those who are overweight, only slight weight loss is linked to delaying — or preventing — diabetes;

More Birthday Candles

It's no secret that people of normal weight are at a higher risk of disease and therefore live longer. But do you know for how long? The risk of death rises by around 30 percent for every 33 pounds of excess weight. The lifetime of an obese person (anyone with a BMI of 40-45) is up to 10 years less than that of a normal-weight person.

How To Keep A Regular Weight

Many factors can influence your weight, including biology, age, gender, diet, family and community, sleep, and even where you live and work. Some of these aspects can make it difficult to lose weight or to keep weight off.

But being busy and eating healthy foods has health benefits for everyone, regardless of age or weight. It is essential to choose nutrient-dense foods and to be active for at least 150 minutes per week. In the thumb rule:

- To maintain your weight the same, you need to consume the same amount of calories as you eat and drink.
- To lose weight, consume more calories than you eat and drink.
- To gain weight, consume fewer calories than you eat and drink.

Maintenance For RegularWeight

Reduce portion size to monitor calorie intake.

Add healthy snacks throughout the day if you want to get more weight.

Physically active as you can be.

Talk to your doctor about your weight, whether you find you weigh too much or too little.

Therefore, being healthy will help you live longer, reduce your chances of developing chronic disease, and help you get more out of your life.

Chapter 16:
14-Day Intermittent Fasting Recipes

BROWNIE CHEESECAKE

Brownie cheesecake is a combination of cheesecake (low in carbohydrate) and brownies that are gluten-free. So it is two delicious desserts in one! The amount of carb in this is less than 0.5g per serving.

Ingredients

Almond flour or coconut flour (that is finely ground)

Butter (soft): grass-fed butter should be used because it contains more healthy fats (omega 3 fatty acids) and has a higher micronutrient level than regular butter. Also to make the butter soft, keep the butter for about 40 minutes at room temperature. This helps to loosen the consistency of the butter and make it soft.

Erythritol (the powdered form): this sweetener is used in keto desserts because it is keto diet friendly as it does not raise the blood sugar level and it is very safe to use.

Cocoa powder: Dutch baking cocoa powder): it is used because just a small amount is needed to achieve a great chocolate taste and flavor and helps to achieve a low carbohydrate recipe.

Vanilla extract (that is free of sugar)

Cream cheese (the full-fat type)

Some chocolate bars (to be grated)

Tools/ Utensils Used

Fridge/ freezer

Parchment paper to line the silicone molds

Mixing bowls

Big spoon

Greater

Silicone molds

Preparation

For The Brownie Layer

Mix the Dutch baking cocoa powder and the vanilla extract in a mixing bowl until it has combined well

Add the soft butter and mix well. (be sure to make the butter mix well in the mixture to form a paste)

Pour the mixture(the brownie layer) halfway into an appropriate silicon mold of the desired size (be sure to fill it halfway so as to allow for the cheese layer to also be poured in it)

The brownie layer can be stored in a fridge pending the time the cheesecake layer would be ready.

For The Cheese Cake Layer

Add the rest of the butter, the almond flour or coconut flour, the rest of the vanilla essence into a mixing bowl and mix till it is very smooth.

When it is very smooth, pour the mixture into the cooled half-filled silicone mold until it is filled up.

Freeze in a freezer for about 2 hours or till it is hard enough.

Remove the already made brownie cheesecake from the silicone mold carefully and serve.

PEANUT BUTTER MOLTEN LAVA CAKE

Nutrition Content In A Serving (One Medium-Sized Cake)

Total Calories: 387 Calories

Calories from fat: 315 Calories

Total Fat: 35.02g

Cholesterol : 215 mg

Protein:10.44g

Carbohydrate:6.41

Fiber: 1.13g

Serving size: 4 servings (4 cakes)

Preparation Time: 25 minutes

Ingredients

2 very big eggs and their yolks

A cup of peanut butter

Chocolate sauce (that is low carb)

Six full tablespoons of almond flour

one full tablespoon of vanilla essence

two tablespoons of coconut oil

seven tablespoons of sweetener (powdered form)

a spoon of butter to grease the baking pan

Tools/ Utensils Needed

oven

baking pan

mixing bowls

a bowl that is microwave safe

spoons

knife

Preparation

Heat the oven to about 370F

Use the butter to grease the baking pan very well so that the cake would remove smoothly without any dent.

Put the peanut butter and coconut oil into a bowl that is microwave safe and stir.

Heat them for a little while to get it melted. When the mixture is already melted, stir it well till it mixes together and is smooth.

Add the powdered sweetener into the melted mixture and whisk it. Also add the almond flour, the vanilla essence, the eggs, and their yolks. Whisk together until the mixture is very smooth.

Fill the baking pan with the batter and bake for about 15 minutes.

Once done, remove the cake from the pan using a knife to loosen the cake from the baking pan.

Place on a serving plate and drizzle it with the chocolate sauce(that is low in carbohydrate)

Follow this process for the four cakes

ITALIAN CREAM CAKE

This cake isn't really Italian as the name implies, never the less it is a great cake that is delicious and also yummy.

Serving size: 4 portions

Preparation Time:

Ingredients

For The Cake

Two cups of almond flour

One cup of coconut flour

One cup of softened butter that is unsalted

4 very big eggs

1 cup of erythritol

A pinch of salt

2 tablespoons of baking powder

One cup of heavy cream

Half tablespoon of cream of tartar

One tablespoon of vanilla extract

One cup of pecans (already chopped)

One cup of already shredded coconut

For The Frosting

Half cup of heavy cream

One cup of soft butter that is unsalted

Two tablespoons of vanilla extract

One cup of cream cheese

Half cup of swerve (powdered)

For The Garnish

Two tablespoons of pecans that are chopped already

Two tablespoons of shredded coconut that are toasted

Tools/ Utensils

Oven

Cake baking pan

Parchment paper liner

Mixing bowl

Preparation

Before starting the preparation, first, heat the oven to about 350F

Use the parchment paper lining to line the inside of the cake baking pan and grease it with a little butter for easy remover

Add the flour, the baking powder, the salt, and the pecans and coconut into a large bowl and stir.

In another bowl, put the sweetener and the butter and cream it until it becomes very fluffy and light.

Remove the yolks from the egg and beat them. Then add to the mixture of sweetener and butter and mix it well.

Then add the heavy cream and the vanilla to the above mixture and mix it very well again.

Add the dry ingredients (the almond flour, the coconut flour, the salt, and the baking powder) into the mixed butter mixture and stir until it is fully combined.

Put the egg whites of the already removed yolk into a bowl and whisk it together with the cream of tartar. Mix it well until it foams.

Then fold this mixture into the already mixed barter. To make the barter light, be sure to fold the egg white mixture lightly.

Pour the batter into the baking pans and bake for about 40 minutes in the already heated oven. By this time, the edges of the cake should be a shade of golden brown and the center of the cake should be firm.

Leave it in the baking pans to cool.

Remove the cake from the pans when they are already cool.

For The Frosting

Put the cream cheese and the butter together in a mixing bowl and start to mix them until the mixture becomes very fluffy and light.

To the mixture, add the sweetener and the vanilla and mix it by beating the mixture.

Next, add the heavy cream to the mixture. To get your desired consistency, add the heavy cream slowly so as to be able to stop when it reaches the desired consistency.

Paste the top of the cake and the side of the cake with the frosting.

On the top layer of the cake, sprinkle the roasted coconut that was shredded and use it to decorate the cake.

GOOEY BUTTER CAKE

Gooey butter cake originated from the United States, from St Louis, Missouri to be precise. The cake is usually dense and flat and also, it usually has a topping of a gooey filling that is sweet and made from butter and cream cheese. The gooey butter cake has three portions: the cake portion, the filling portion, and the sprinkling portion. The cake portion is made with a cake mix that is boxed with a lot of added butter, the addition of lesser eggs, and also no addition of liquids to the cake batter. This is done like that so that it will not rise too much and also so that it will remain buttery and dense. The filling is made by mixing butter, granulated sugar, cream cheese, and egg together by beating it together. Then this mixture is over the top of the cake and then baked till the filling gets gooey. The sprinkling portion is made by sprinkling a desired amount of sugar (or sweetener of choice) on the cake.

Nutrition Content

Total Calories: 268 calories

Calories from fat: 218 calories

Fat: 24. 2 g

Carbohydrates: 4.2 g

Protein: 6.1 g

Fiber: 1.6 g

Portion size: 15 servings

Preparation Time: 60 minutes

Ingredients

For The Cake

Two cups of coconut flour (or almond flour))

One egg

A little salt

Half cup of swerve sweetener

One tablespoon of vanilla extract

Two tablespoons of baking powder

Half cup of butter that is already melted

Two tablespoons of whey protein powder that is not flavored.

For the filling portion

Two cups of already softened cream cheese

One tablespoon of vanilla extract

A cup of powdered swerve sweetener

Two eggs

For The Sprinkling Portion

A cop of powdered swerve sweetener

Tools / Utensils Needed

Oven

Baking pan

Mixing bowls

Stirrer

Preparation

For The Cake Portion

Before starting the preparation process, heat the oven to about 325F

Grease the inside of the baking pan to be used. Grease it with butter to make the cake remove easily.

Put the almond /coconut flour, the baking powder, a little salt, the protein powder and the sweetener in a mixing bowl and mix together until it combines. Also, add the egg, the vanilla extract and the butter and mix well till it combines evenly with the mixture. Pour this mixture into the previously greased baking pan halfway.

For The Filling

Mix the butter and cream cheese together in another mixing bowl and mix well by beating them together. Then add the sweetener until it has fully dissolved and combined with the mixture, then add the eggs and vanilla essence till it is very smooth.

Pour the filling mixture into the half-filled baking pan and bake for about 45 minutes. By this time, the edges of the cake are golden brown in color and the center is still jiggling.

Remove the cake from the baking pan and allow cooling. Then remove and place in a serving plate.

Dust or sprinkle the cake with the powdered swerve and cut the cake into equal bars.

PECAN PIE CHEESECAKE

Nutrition Content

Total Calories: 340 calories

Calories from Fat: 279 calories

Fat: 31.03 g

Protein: 5.89 g

Carbohydrate: 4.97 g

Fiber 1.42 g

Serving size: 10 servings

Preparation time: 50 minutes +3 hours to chill

Ingredients

For The Crust

A cup of almond flour

A little salt

Two tablespoons of swerve sweetener in the powdered form

Two tablespoons of melted butter

For The Topping

Two tablespoons of butter

One tablespoon of whipping cream (heavy)

Half a cup of already powdered swerve sweetener

Two tablespoons of yacon syrup

Toasted pecans (whole) to garnish the cake

One tablespoon of vanilla extract or caramel extract

For The Cheese Cake Filling

Half cup of whipping cream (heavy)

One big egg

Half tablespoon of vanilla extract

Two cups of softened cream cheese

Five tablespoons of powdered swerve sweeteners

Preparation

For The Crust

Add the almond flour, the salt and the swerve sweetener into a big mixing bowl and whisk together.

Add the melted butter and stir well until the mixture becomes clumpy.

Put the mixture into a springform pan and press it to the bottom and up the sides of the baking pan. Keep in the freezer during the time to prepare the pecan pie filling.

Pecan Pie Filling

Melt the butter. This can be done by putting it in a small pot and placing it over low heat. Add the yacon syrup and the sweetener into the melted butter and mix it together until they have combined evenly. Add the vanilla extract or chocolate extract and the heavy whipping cream and stir until they have combined fully.

Then add the egg and start to cook it until this mixture gets thick. After about a minute, stop cooking the mixture from the heat and add the salt and pecan and then stir well.

Spread the mixture over the crust's bottom.

For The Cheese Cake Filling

Put the cream cheese into a bowl and beat it until it becomes smooth. Then add the sweetener, the whipping cream, the vanilla extract, and the egg, beating each ingredient as you add each one.

Pour this mixture on the pecan pie filling and make sure it spreads to the edges.

For The Baking

Use a big piece of foil paper to warp the bottom of the springform baking pan. On top of the springform baking pan, out a piece of towel (paper). Be careful not to let it touch the cheesecake. Also, wrap the foil paper around the top of the pan. The essence of wrapping with foil paper is to prevent excess moisture from entering into the cake batter.

Bake the cake in an oven for few minutes and remove the cake from the baking pan and let it cool down. After this, place the cooled cake in the refrigerator and refrigerate it for over 3 hours.

For The Topping

Place a small pot over low heat; put the butter in it to get it melted. Then put the yacon syrup and the sweetener, whisk them to make the mixture combine well, then add the vanilla or caramel extract, stir, also add the heavy whipping cream and stir again.

Drizzle this mixture (the topping) on the cheesecake and use the toasted pecans to garnish it.

CARAMEL CAKE

This cake is basically a vanilla flavored cake that is almond flour-based.

Nutritional Content

Total Calories: 388 calories

Calories from Fat: 314 calories

Fat: 34. 9 g

Protein:9.5 g

Carbohydrate: 7.6 g

Fiber: 3.4 g

Serving Size: 3 servings

Preparation Time: 1 hour 10 minutes

Ingredients

One cup of almond flour

Three tablespoons of coconut flour

Half a cup of almond milk

Three tablespoons of already softened butter

Two tablespoons of whey protein flour(the unflavored one)

A big egg

A cup of caramel source that does not have sugar

A pinch of salt

Half tablespoon of baking powder

Half tablespoon of the vanilla extract

Preparation

To Make The Cake

First of all, heat the ovens to about 375F. Take a baking pan and grease it to avoid the cake getting stuck in it during removal. Place the parchment paper in the baking pan and also grease the parchment paper.

Mix the flours (the almond flour and the coconut flour) in a mixing bowl and whisk in the baking powder, salt, and whey protein.

In another mixing bowl, whisk the sweetener and the eggs together. Stop when the mixture becomes fluffy and white. Beat the butter into the mixture and also beat the vanilla extract in too.

Add the rest of the ingredients into the barter. Remember to beat the mixture very well upon the addition of an ingredient.

Pour the batter into the cake baking pan and let it spread to the edges of the baking pan. Make sure the top of the batter is smoothened and place the baking pan in the oven.

Bake the cake till the color of the edges are golden in color and also till the top of the cake becomes firm. This should take about 25 minutes.

Remove the cake from the baking pan and put it in a flat plate for it to cool down. Remove the parchment paper longing if it sticks to the cake.

KENTUCKY BUTTER CAKE

This type of cake is moist and also contains a butter cake plus a butter sauce that is very sweet and soaks the cake. The major ingredient in this cake is butter. A very large amount of butter is needed to make this cake. The difference between the normal Kentucky butter cake and the keto version is the type of flour used. In the keto version, almond flour is used as against the wheat flour used in the normal version.

Nutrition content of a serving

Total calories: 301 calories

Calories from fat: 244 calories

Fat: 27.07 g

Carbohydrate: 5.54 g

Protein: 7.34 g

Fiber: 2.4 g

Serving Size: 4 servings

Preparation time: 1 hour 30 minutes

Ingredients

For The Cake

One cup of almond flour

Three tablespoons of coconut flavor

A little water

Half cup of soft butter(make the butter soft by placing at room temperature for some time)

2 eggs

Two tablespoons of protein powder

One tablespoon of vanilla extract

One tablespoon of baking powder

Three tablespoons of whipped cream

A pinch of salt

Four tablespoons of granulated swerve sweetener

For The Butter Glaze

Two tablespoons of butter

Half tablespoon of water

A quarter cup of granulated swerve sweetener

Half tablespoon of vanilla essence

For The Garnishing

One tablespoon of swerve sweetener

Preparation

For The Cake

Preheat an oven to about 350F, get a cake baking pan, add a little butter to it and grease the pan with the butter, then put two tablespoons of almond flour in the pan and dust it with the flour.

Put the dry ingredients (the almond flour, the baking powder, the salt, the coconut flour, and the protein powder) in a bowl and mix them together.

Get another bowl and beat the Swerve sweetener and the butter together until the mixture turns fluffy and very light. Add the vanilla extract and egg to the mixture and beat it together.

Add the first mixture (the almond flour mixture) to the butter mixture and beat together. Then add the whipping cream and the water to the mixture and beat well until it combines very well.

Pour the batter into the already greased and dusted baking pan. Bake it until it becomes firm and the color changes to a golden brown color. This should take about an hour.

For The Butter Glaze

Place a medium saucepan on medium heat, put the butter and the swerve sweetener in the saucepan and let them melt together. Mix this mixture well to make it combine. Also, add the vanilla extract and the water and whisk them well until the mixture is fully combined.

Create holes in the cake in the baking pan. This can be done with a skewer.

Pour the butter glaze on the cake in the baking pan while it is still warm and let the cake with the butter glaze get cooled down in the pan.

Remove the cake from the baking pan and put it on a serving plate. Be careful to use a knife to make the sides of the cake get loosened so as to make the whole of the cake remove without any dents.

While the cake is on the serving plate, use the powdered swerve sweetener to dust the top and the sides of the cake.

The cake is ready to be served. You can serve with sweetened whipped cream and/or fresh strawberries.

TEXAS CHEESECAKE

It is not restricted to the Americans alone as the name implies. It is consumed all over the world and is a great dessert on the keto diet list.

Nutritional Content

Total Calories: 230 calories

Calories from fat: 183 calories

Fat: 20.3 g

Carbohydrate: 5.9 g

Protein: 5.8 g

Fiber: 3.1 g

Serving Size: 4 servings

Preparation Time: 45 minutes

Ingredients

For The Cake

Half a cup of almond flour

Two tablespoons of coconut flour

One tablespoon of swerve sweetener

Half tablespoon of baking powder

One tablespoon of protein powder that is not flavored

Three tablespoons of salt

A pinch of salt

Two tablespoons of water

Two tablespoons of whipping cream

One egg

Two tablespoons of cocoa powder

For The Frosting

Two tablespoons of pecans that are already chopped

Two tablespoons of butter

A little water (about two tablespoons)

Three tablespoons of cocoa powder

One heaped tablespoon of whipping cream

One teaspoon of vanilla extract

Half a cup of swerve sweetener (in the powdered form)

One teaspoon of xanthan gum

Preparation

For The Cake

First of all heat the oven to about 325F before starting the preparation of the cake.

Get a sheet pan (rimmed, about 10 by 15 inches), grease it with butter.

Mix the coconut flour, the almond flour, baking powder, sweetener, salt, and protein powder by whisking it in a mixing bowl. Make sure there are no lumps in the mixture.

Melt the cocoa powder and powder; add a little water till it is fully melted. Do this by putting the cocoa powder and butter in a small pot and place over low heat. When this melted mixture is boiling, remove it and pour it into the mixing bowl with the whisked dry ingredients.

Add the vanilla extract, the eggs, a little water, and cream. Stir them in until they have fully combined together

Pour the batter in a baking pan and spread it in it.

Place in the preheated oven and bake it for about 20 minutes. By this time, the cake should be firm already.

For The Frosting

Put the cocoa powder, the butter, vanilla extract and a little water in a small saucepan. Place it on medium heat and boil it till it simmers. Stir it to make it smooth. Add the vanilla extract and the sweetener (in powdered form) a little at a time and stir it while adding each portion. If there are any clumps in the mixture, stir and whisk it well to make the clumps dissolve.

Add xanthan gum to the declumped mixture and whisk it very well.

Pour the frost on the cake while still warm and sprinkle pecans on the cake. Let the cake cool for about an hour (so as to make the frosting get set)

Serve

CINNAMON ROLL COFFEE CAKE

This keto cake is filled with cinnamon and glazed with cream cheese that is sugar- free. It is gluten-free and also low in carbohydrates.

Nutritional Content In A Serving

Total calories: 222 calories

Calories from fat: 174 calories

Fat: 19.3 g

Protein: 7.2 g

Carbohydrate: 5.4 g

Serving size: 4 portions (a small-sized cake)

Preparation time: 50 minutes

Ingredients

For The Cake

1 cup of almond flour

A quarter tablespoon of already melted butter

A quarter tablespoon of almond milk

A quarter cup of swerve sweetener

Half tablespoon of vanilla extract

1 egg

A pinch of salt

Two tablespoons of protein powder that is unflavored

A quarter tablespoon of baking powder

For The Cinnamon Filling

One tablespoon of cinnamon in the ground form

One tablespoon of Swerve sweetener in the powdered form

For The Cream Cheese Frosting

A quarter tablespoon of vanilla extract

A quarter tablespoon of swerve sweetener

One tablespoon of cheese cream that is already softened

A quarter tablespoon of heavy whipping cream.

Preparation

Get a small baking pan and grease it with butter

Heat the oven to 325F

Put the ground cinnamon in a small mixing bowl and add the swerve sweetener, then mix it very well. When it has mixed well enough, leave it and start to prepare the cake.

Add all the dry ingredients for the cake in a large bowl. This includes the almond flour, the salt, the protein, the baking powder, and sweetener. Mix them well by whisking them together.

Add the already melted butter, the eggs, almond milk, and vanilla extract and stir vigorously as you add the ingredients for easy and thorough combination.

Put about half of the batter into the greased baking pan and spread it. Then add more than half of the prepared cinnamon filling into the baking pan and add the remaining batter on top of the cinnamon filling. Spread it with a spatula.

Bake until the top of the cake is golden brown in color. This should take about 35 minutes.

Remove the cake into a serving plate and let it get cool.

Add cream, cream cheese, vanilla extract, and the powdered erythritol into a bowl and mix together in a small bowl to make the frosting. Beat the mixture well until it is well combined and smooth.

Pipe the frosting on the cooled cake.

PEANUT BUTTER MUG CAKE

It is important to work through the preparation of the peanut butter mug cake quickly because peanut butter thickens the cake batter the longer it waits.

Nutrition Value Of A Serving (One Mug Cake)

Total calories: 210 calories

Calories from fat: 160 calories

Fat: 17.8 g

Protein: 6.4 g

Fiber : 3 g

Serving size: 5 portions (5 mug cakes)

Preparation time: 5 minutes

Ingredients

A quarter cup of peanut butter

A quarter cup of butter

Half cup of almond flour

3 tablespoons of chocolate chips that are sugar-free

Half a tablespoon of vanilla extract

A quarter cup of swerve sweetener

One tablespoon of baking powder

A little water

Two eggs

Preparation

Put the peanut butter and the butter in a bowl that is microwave safe and place in the microwave to melt it. Make use of the melted mixture is smooth.

Put the almond flour, the sweetener and the baking powder in a bowl and mix together by whisking it. Add the melted peanut butter and butter mixture, the eggs, vanilla extract, and a little water and stir it well till it combines. Also, add the chocolate chips and stir them.

Divide the batter into 5 mugs and bake in the microwave for about a minute each. It should be puff and set by this time.

The cake is ready to be served, serve hot

GINGERBREAD CAKE ROLL

Nutrition Value Of A Serving

Calories: 206 calories

Calories from fat: 163 g

Fat: 18.06 g

Protein: 5.68 g

Carbohydrate: 3.99g

Serving size: 4 servings

Preparation Time: 60 minutes

Ingredients

For The Cake

Half cup of almond flour

One tablespoon of ethical approval

A quarter cup of a powdered sweetener

Half tablespoon of grass fed gelatin

One-eighth tablespoon of cream of tartar

A quarter tablespoon of powdered ginger

A pinch of salt

A little cinnamon powder

A quarter tablespoon of vanilla extract

One eight of powdered cloves

One large egg

For The Vanilla Cream Filling

One cup of softened cream cheese

Half cup of whipping cream

Two tablespoons of powdered sweetener

A quarter tablespoon of vanilla extract

Preparation

For The Cake

Heat the oven to 350F before starting the cake preparation process. Place a parchment paper in a baking pan and line the baking pan with it. Use a little butter to grease the sides of the baking pan and also the parchment paper.

Whisk the almond flour, the cocoa powder, the powdered sweetener, ginger, gelatin, powdered cloves together in a medium mixing bowl.

Get another mixing bowl and mix the granulated sugar together with the egg yolk until the mixture gets thickened and the color turns light yellow.

Also, add the vanilla extract and beat the mixture well.

Beat the egg whites and the cream of tartar and a little salt together in another mixing bowl until the mixture becomes frothy. When it is already frothy, add the remaining sweetener and beat it well.

Fold the beaten egg yolks into the beaten egg whites gently. Then fold this into the almond flour mixture. Be careful not to make it deflated.

Make the batter spread into the already greased baking pan and bake for 12 minutes until it springs back when the top is touched.

Remove it from the oven and let it get cooled a little before removing it. You can remove it by using a knife to make the edges loosen. Cover the cake with another piece of parchment paper and also use a kitchen towel to cover it. Put another baking sheet that is large on top of it and flip the cake over.

Peel the parchment paper gently from the cake and also roll up the kitchen towel gently and let the cake cool down.

For The Vanilla Cream Filling

Beat half of the whipping cream with the cream cheese in a mixing bowl. Beat it till it becomes smooth.

Beat the remaining whipping cream and the sweetener in a big mixing bowl. Then add the vanilla extract and the mixture of the whipping cream and beat very well, but do not overbeat it. Keep about half of the mixture to decorate the cake.

Unroll the cake carefully. Let the cake curl up on the ends and do not lay it down flat completely.

Spread the rest of the filling on the cake and roll it up back gently. Do not roll it up back with the kitchen towel.

Place it on a serving plate. Place the seam side down.

Put the remaining cream mixture on the center of the cake in different shapes. You can use an icing pipe to achieve desired shapes.

Keep In the refrigerator.

KETO PUMPKIN CHEESECAKE

Nutrition Value Of A Serving

Total calories: 246 g

Calories from fat: 211 g

Fat: 23. 4 g

Protein: 5.3 g

Carbohydrates: 3.23 g

Fiber: 1.1 g

Serving size: 4 servings

Preparation Time: 55 minutes + chill time

Ingredients

For The Crust

A quarter cup of almond flour

Half tablespoon of melted butter

One tablespoon of powdered sweetener

A pinch of salt

A quarter tablespoon of powdered ginger

A quarter tablespoon of cinnamon powder

For The Pumpkin Cheese Cake

A cup of softened cheese

One egg

Half a cup of softened cream cheese

Half tablespoon of pumpkin pie spice

Three tablespoons of pumpkin puree

Half tablespoon of vanilla extract

Preparation

For The Crust

Whisk the almond flour, the spices, salt, and the sweetener together in a big mixing bowl. Add the melted butter and stir until the mixture becomes clumpy.

Pour the mixture into a springform baking pan.

For The Filing

Beat the softened cheese and the cream cheese together until it combines well. Add the sweetener and stir well until it becomes smooth.

Add the pumpkin pie spice, pumpkin puree, the vanilla extract and combine it well by beating it well. Add the egg and continue beating it until it combines well.

Use a large foil paper to wrap the bottom of the springform pan. Wrap it tightly. Put a paper towel over the pan. Be careful not to make it touch the cake. Then wrap another foil over the cake top. The reason for wrapping with foil is to prevent excess moisture from entering the cake.

Bake the cake for about 30 minutes; bring it to cool it down.

Refrigerate for about four hours. When it is chilled, use a knife to remove the cake.

If you like, you can add a topping of caramel sauce and whipped cream

CANNOLI SHEET CAKE

Nutrition Value Of A Serving

Total calories: 235 calories

Calories from fat: 180 calories

Fat: 20 g

Protein: 6.8 g

Carbohydrates: 6.2 g

Calcium : 2.9 mg

Serving size: 5 servings

Preparation Time: 40 minutes

Ingredients

For The Sheet Cake

Half cup of almond flour

Half tablespoon of vanilla extract

A quarter cup of sweetener

A little water

Two tablespoons of coconut flour

Three tablespoons of melted butter

Two tablespoons of protein powder

One egg

A pinch of salt

Half tablespoon of baking powder

For The Cannoli Cream Frosting

A quarter cup of milk ricotta

Two tablespoons of chocolate chips (sugar-free)

Two tablespoons of softened cheese cream

A quarter tablespoon of vanilla extract

A quarter cup of powdered sweetener

A quarter cup of heavy whipping cream

Preparation

Heat the oven to about 325F. Grease a small jelly roll pan to avoid the cake sticking to the bottom of the pan.

Whisk the almond flour, coconut flour, sweetener, protein powder, baking powder, and the salt in a big mixing bowl. Add the, already melted butter, eggs, water, and the vanilla extract and stir until they have combined very well.

Pour the batter in the already prepared baking pan and spread it so that there is an even distribution of the batter in the baking pan. Bake the bake for about 22 minutes till the color becomes golden brown and becomes firm while touching.

Remove the baking pan from the oven and let cool completely.

COCONUT FLOUR CHOCOLATE CUPCAKE

Nutritional Value Of A Serving

Total Calories: 268 calories

Calories from fat:

Serving Size: 4 servings (4 cupcakes)

Preparation Time: 35 minutes

Ingredients

Four tablespoons of melted butter

Three tablespoons of cocoa butter

Three tablespoons of almond cream that is unsweetened

Two eggs

A pinch of salt

Three tablespoons of sweetener

One tablespoon of baking powder

One tablespoon of vanilla essence

For The Butter Cream

Half cup of sweetener

One tablespoon of instant coffee

Two tablespoons of softened cream cheese

A little hot water

Half a cup of whipping cream

Preparation

For The Cup Cakes

Heat the oven to 370 F

Use parchment paper to line the inside of the muffin tin

Add the cocoa powder, melted butter, the espresso powder, and melted butter together in a big mixing bowl and whisk them together.

Add the vanilla essence and eggs to the mixture then add the baking powder, coconut flour, a pinch of salt and the sweetener, and then beat well to combine it together.

CONCLUSION

Intermittent fasting is a lifestyle that is not only easy and healthy but also enjoys a meal. Although it opposes many of today's views and ideas, there is the evidence behind it. With all these new ideas and diets, you'd think the world would be getting more fit instead of fat at an all-time high. Through research and science, it proves IF works, and if the Romans, the height of fitness, used it to stay fit, why shouldn't we?

Intermittent fasting was successful for short-term weight loss in healthy, overweight, and obese people. Randomized controlled trials with a long-term follow-up duration are needed to ensure commitment to the diet and long-term retention of weight loss without regaining lost weight. Future studies should also include specific population subgroups, such as people with cardiovascular risk factors and type 2 diabetes mellitus, as these patients are more likely to benefit from weight loss that may influence the disease process. In summary, obesity and overweight are an international health issue, and measures such as ADF are needed to help people achieve weight loss.

Now you know what IF is and how it can help you lose weight quickly, comfortably, and seamlessly.

It also involves cycles of starvation, which places the body in a state of fat burning. During the fasting time (usually 16 hours), there are improvements in the body that facilitate increased longevity, cellular regeneration, reduced inflammation, and changes in hormonal body weight regulation. Although it is not suitable for those who are insulin-dependent who require regular meals, intermittent fasting can be reasonably easy to adapt and can be a proper diet for many individuals.

Although this is a "diet," it does not necessarily mean that anyone who practices an intermittent fasting diet is using it to lose weight. Although, indeed, this diet may allow some patients to break through weight-loss plateaus, it also provides a variety of other health benefits and may be helpful for some health conditions.

INTERMITTENT FASTING FOR WOMEN

The Ultimate Step-By-Step Guide to Meal Planning for The Burning of Fat, Slow Aging, and Regulation of Physiological Functions Through Metabolic Autophagy

By

Asuka Young

Introduction

It is not in your head, ladies—when it comes to weight, men and women don't live in an equal world. Men claim to have a faster metabolism, with their bigger bodies and larger muscles and bones. Girls put on weight during puberty, and boys put on muscle. Females need more fat than men from fertilization to breastfeeding. While you read, be mindful that while the odds seem to stack against us, we can conquer stubborn fat and boost our forms and wellbeing — first a quick description of women's fat-burning problems and then the tools to conquer them.

In today of today, weight loss and diet, no word can generate more anxiety, anger, and confusion than fasting. The word evokes fantasies that people are hungry for weeks and days without a food bite and only drink fruit juices. A conventional fast is problematic and perhaps even unsafe for some people, but intermittent fasting relies on the new calory loss research.

Various methods can accomplish weight loss. A diet and exercise combination works best. If you cannot lose weight or hold it away, particularly if you suffer from related health problems like diabetes, you can find the relief you need in surgery.

Chapter One:
Intermittent Fasting For Women

Intermittent fasting may seem like a great choice for women who are interested in weight loss, but many want to know that women can fast? Is intermittent fasting for women effective? Several key studies have been conducted on intermittent fasting that can help clarify this interesting new dietary trend.

Intermittent fasting is also known as alternative fasting, although this diet certainly varies. A new study was carried out by the American Journal of Clinical Nutrition in which 16 obese men and women engaged in a 10-week program. During the fasting days, participants ate up to 25% of their estimated energy requirements. They received nutritional advice for the rest of the time but were not given a certain guideline during this time.

As predicted, participants lost weight as a result of this research, but some specific changes were exciting. The people were still all obese after only ten weeks, but cholesterol, LDL cholesterol, triglycerides, and systolic blood pressure had changed. What made this interesting finding was that most people have to lose weight before seeing the same changes than these study participants. It was a surprising discovery that inspired many to pursue fasting.

Intermittent fasting has beneficial effects on women. With women who are trying to lose weight, women must have a much greater proportion of fat in their bodies. The body mostly takes fat to the carbohydrate storage for the first 6 hours when it tries to lose weight. Women who practice a healthy diet and workout will combat stubborn fat, but fasting is a realistic solution.

Intermittent Fasting for women More than 50 Of course, as we hit menopause, our bodies and metabolism shift. One of the main shifts of women in over 50 years are that they have a slower metabolism and become weighty. Fasting may be a safe way to reverse this weight gain and avoid it. Research has shown that this method of fasting helps to control appetite, and people who regularly observe it do not feel the same hunger as others. Intermittent quicking will allow you to avoid eating too much on a daily basis when you are over 50, and you are trying to adapt to your slower metabolism.

Once you reach 50, the body frequently develops chronic diseases, such as high cholesterol and hypertension. Intermittent rapidity, both cholesterol and blood pressure have reduced, even without significant weight loss. When you find that your numbers increase every year at the doctor's office, you may be able to bring them back down without losing a lot of weight.

For each woman, intermittent fasting may not be a great idea. Anyone with a certain health condition or who is normally hypoglycemic should consult a doctor. But this current dietary pattern has specific advantages for women who naturally store more fat in their bodies and may have difficulty getting rid of fat shops.

Fat Burning Secrets for Women

Distribution of body fat
Women carry about twice as much body fat as men, mainly to help them carry babies and feed them. Fat is the main source of energy required for the production and safety of fetuses. They don't know where the fat cells expand and shrink.

The fat cells in the lower body, in which women tend to put inches, are more vulnerable to fat storage. The upper body fat cells, in which men tend to carry extra weight, are more likely to release fat. Women who died know that body fat begins to melt off the upper body as they lose weight, first followed by persevering lower body fat.

Furthermore, the reverse is true for weight increases. The fat cells in the breasts, thighs, ass, and abdomen are first swollen. Women who died of yoyo for years have an upper body, which is comparatively smaller than their lower body.

Hormones

Hormones promote water retention in fat cells during pregnancy and the menstrual cycle. The excess fluid slows the movement and makes transferring fat much harder.

Within women's bodies, progesterone stimulates appetite and mood. This induces malnutrition in the second half of your menstrual cycle and is responsible for your pregnancy's ravenous appetite. Progesterone also makes you less likely to exercise and sleepiness. Women taking birth control pills gain 3 to 5 pounds as a side effect on average.

Pregnancy

Pregnancy Fat cells in a woman's body not only grow but often multiply during pregnancy. After the pregnancy is over, the fat cells remain and are prepared to expand when the body takes in more calories than it consumes. The thyroid gland that controls the metabolism also becomes extremely lenient during pregnancy to help keep the body healthy. Not surprisingly, the weight loss problem may be compounded after two or three children.

Menopause

Women start developing less estrogen, a defensive hormone, during peri-menopause (10 years prior to menopause). We also start sleeping less, and our appetite is increased. As a result of peri-menopause, the fat tends to build up around the tail and chest, increasing our heart disease risk.

Aging

Each decade, women begin to lose an average of about 7 pounds of muscle mass in the middle of the '20s (compared to 5 pounds for men). To make matters worse, women who do not exercise tend to receive 1-2 pounds of fat a year—for their lives. And the amount of fat gains can be much higher depending on the lifestyle.

And you probably lost about 15 pounds of healthy aerobic muscle in your mid-40s, replacing it with more than lethargic overweight 20 pounds-and this was conservative! Your metabolism has slowed dramatically, and your body composition has shifted unfavorably.

To make matters worse, you have accelerated the muscle loss process if you have dieted (I imagine you tried one or two). Exercise without Dieting can lead to a muscle loss of 28% to 25%.

Aging also makes it harder to hide excess fat. As the skin starts losing the elasticity and sluggishness, it has a longer period of time holding fat cells and is often known when cellulite.

Why do men have it easier

Why do men have it easier to stimulate bone and muscle development? We don't lose testosterone so easily that we lack estrogen. Men have more muscle, have more bone minerals, and eat around 35% more calories than women. Men also respond to training more quickly.

While men do not usually live as long as women, they begin and end with more bone, muscle, and testosterone than women. When a woman is 60 years old, her body probably contains 20 to 30 pounds of muscle—IF she doesn't function.

Women also face many social and emotional challenges that can make them a slave to their level; resist exercises in fear of spot reductions and quick fixes; such doubts, prejudices, and bugaboos, which keep so many women hostage, can easily fill a book, but let us skip it and discuss solutions that DO. Women also face many social and emotional challenges.

Now that you understand the unique physiological challenges that women are faced with, let's talk about how to conquer them in order to achieve the solid, fit body you want.

The secret to fat-burning is exercise. When you do one thing, use the following ten tips to integrate 2-3 strength and cardio routines into your weekly routine. The outcome is guaranteed!

Here are my top ten women's fat-burning secrets.

1. Warming up before a strength exercise–warming up increases muscle movement by approximately 55%, which enhances muscle contracture. You'll sweat faster, so you can regulate the temperature of your body. It also begins the neuromuscular link that activates the release of carbohydrates and fatty enzymes and hormones and decreases the perceived exercise during strength training. This requirement can only be fulfilled by 5 minutes walking or cycling.

2. Diversify your cardiovascular preparation-Alter two or more cardiovascular behaviors like walking and cycling or kickboxing and step-aerobics. It helps to develop cardiovascular fitness optimally, and retains the fun element of exercise, helps to prevent overwork and injury. In the end, you're going to spend more calories.

3. Integrate various exercise methods-use a mix of continuous training, sprint, circuit, and pace play (Fartlek). Modification of techniques causes your body to adapt and become more successful. Vary the severity and change the types of effects. For example, if you walk the same path every day at the same pace, start to introduce accelerated splashes intermittently. The idea behind it is that transition keeps the body going, changing, and consuming fat.

4. Plan your training in phases-organize your training in a cyclical system. For example, exercise at a lower intensity for 45-60 minutes for two to three weeks, then exercise at the

maximum intensity for the following two to three weeks. The following 2 to 3 weeks last 30 to 45 minutes at moderate intensity. This program allows you to maintain a high fitness level rather than overtrain. This process of training structures allows your body to make fat burning five more effective. Train Circuit-Perform several enforcement exercises with a short cardiovascular segment. For example, press your legs, pull the side down and crunch the abdominal, and then cycle for 3 minutes. Do three more strength exercises and then walk for 3 minutes. Circuit training has a lower rate of dropout, is an efficient calorie burner, improves muscle strength, and decreases body fat.

6. Multi-Joint Strength Train-choose exercises that function in a compound of muscle groups-that means more than one muscle group at a time. This gives you the most miles per exercise. For example, squats, lunges, and push-ups are included. You need 35-50 calories per day for every pound of muscle in your body, while each pound of fat in your body needs just 2 modest calories a day.

7. Exercise first in the morning-morning exercisers are more likely to appear. Earlier in the day, you can increase the odds of missing your workout with interruptions and exhaustion. Morning exercise also helps to regulate your hormone response to release fat and get your metabolism going.

8. Have a "primary" meal before exercising—it helps to burn fat with a small balanced meal before exercise. The blood sugar will increase when you eat, and exercise will work like insulin to help regulate blood glucose. Eating also gives you the energy to make your workout more intense, so you will burn more calories.

9. Eat 5 to 6 small foods a day — Food has a thermal effect, which means your body needs energy (calories) to digest your food. Eating several times during the day increases the thermal effect so that more calories are consumed. Eating also stops you from thinking that you are deprived of food and prevents malnutrition from happening, which can lead you to binge eating.

10. 10. Train with strength—You have to upgrade from "pink weights" and gentle walking in order to get the full benefit of fitness. Don't think about increasing resistance and testing the muscles and cardiovascular system. To alter, you must move your physical limits beyond what you're used to.

I'll leave you with a hydration bonus tip. In order to metabolize the fat, it must first be released out of the fat cell and then transferred to the liver and other active tissues as fuel through the bloodstream. When you are in a dehydrated state, the liver must support the kidneys and can not concentrate on the task of releasing fat. , you can achieve a female, strong, fit, and younger look, regardless of age or legacy. To a certain degree, you can solve any deficiencies and trouble areas with healthy, symmetrical strength, aerobic and adaptive training, and nutritional food choices.

Concentrate on the best you can be. A streamlined and balanced body is both practical and feasible.

Is It Healthy To Fast?

Let us help you with your research: 80 percent or more of those writing about fasting did not fast for much more than a day or two.

Many of these same writers copied their knowledge from other "experts" whose personal experience was never fasted and who did not know anything about the subject.

The novice writers may typically be identified by their opening statements, which most often consist of positive comments and a leading question. The most famous lead-in seems to be: "Speech has been practiced around the world for hundreds of years... but can this actually help you to avoid illnesses, help you to lose weight, and make you healthier?" The fact is, this is not a technique to be followed; it is a decision to be made.

- Is it a quick and easy thing? Probably not, and on many grounds:
- most Americans have a tradition of eating; most like not eating;
- many are too much food addicted;
- If someone takes a meal, what are they saying?
- What do they say?
- "I am hungriest!"
- Americans are used to eating 24 hours a day in their belly;
- most of them have never listened to the word "fast;"
- those who have heard it believe it is just a religious exercise;
- Those who advocate fasting suggest it only for a few days or advocate fasting with juice instead of water; most of the Web information regarding fasting is negative;
- Most fasting at is negative.
- Is it possible to significantly improve serious medical conditions by fasting?
- Is it safe to fast?
- Can quickness have longevity?
- Weight loss by fasting Is fasting an effective weight loss technique to answer the question?

First, we have to consider what fasting is, what it entails, how our body reacts, and what effects are anticipated over the specific length of the fast.

Some relevant factors to consider:

1. do eating disorders,
2. drug addictions like medications or
3. alcohol affects the subject?
- How is the health of the subject? (They should be under medical supervision if questionable.)

- What is their age? (Parental and or health supervision should be needed for under 18)
- How long is the speed? (It is important to set a fair lower goal.)
- What do you want? (What do they intend physically and mentally to achieve?)
- Do they work quickly? (Home or employed?)
- Do they have their friends and family's support?

These are issues and questions which a healthcare practitioner should bring to the subject and be able to address and respond. Unfortunately, trained and experienced people in this field of health and preventive medicine have a severe shortage.

Eating disorders

The nervous bulimia, anorexia nervosa, and binge eating are characterized by irregular eating habits, which can contribute to either insufficient or excessive eating. These will ultimately lead to severe physical or mental disorders or diseases. Fasting can have very serious consequences for a person with one of these disorders. Individuals with an eating disorder who end up fasting may try to catch all the food they abstained in just a few days during fasting. This experience could worsen you're eating disorder seriously.

Your General Health

Before using rapidly, the general health of the subject should be assessed. Fasting only for a couple of days is rarely a problem, but it can be a problem if you have a junk food diet before. Remember, you shouldn't try a long-term fast if you have serious problems with your kidneys or liver or probably problems with your immune system or taking prescription medicines.

Duration of The Fast

The length of your first short should not be a stressful experience. If you don't feel that you can last longer, continue fasting for two days. Seek three the next week, and so on. This will acclimatize the body and brain to this new experience. You can also try to fast with juice for a few days, then turn to distilled water. My first dinner was for 19 days at age 25, working as the chef and cooking 16 hours a day in my own restaurant. Not everyone can, but start anywhere you can and practice your body a little at a time.

Motivation or hopes

A therapy A quick way to do something becomes better if you are inspired by a target or a dream of what the results are going to be. My reason for fasting was to get rid of a rather rare condition of my foot gout. My dream was that it would happen. It was the worst case my doctor ever saw for someone as young as me. He said that the prescribed 1000 mg Zyloprim would eventually destroy my kidneys. A restaurant customer told me I needed to read Dr. Charles Bragg's two books, The Miracle of Fasting and The Shocking Truth About Food. I noticed the mixture of drinking from 1 to 1/2 gallons a day while fasting could get rid of my gout! This was reason enough for me to stay with it 16 hours a day, despite the temptations.

In 15 days, my taste completely disappeared, and I just stayed for four more days to make sure. For the next 40 + years, I continued drinking 1-1/2 gallons of distilled water every day and fast at least 21 days a year. As a result, in over 40 years, I have never been sick or a doctor or taken medicine for disease! Only a coincidence? I don't think so. I don't think so.

40 Day Fast While Working

Five years ago, I fasted 40 days of distilled water and worked in construction every day. On my thirty-fourth quick day, I wanted to show my crew a sign. And I carried five tons of small rocks in the size of basketballs in a 1 hour by myself to the backyard of a residence on the street. For 34 days, I hadn't eaten food and was 59 years old. Once you quickly do, other major organs will finally rest, and everything that saves vital energy can be used to prepare (digest) food for other things. I feel I have proven my point.

Fasting To Detoxify the Body

Fasting to detoxify the body cannot get rid of toxins if you are undernourished with the right nutrients. they lack the right number of phytochemicals and antioxidants to protect our cells against harm. Toxins and waste are found in cellular tissue; they are called Advanced Glycation Ends (AGE) products that contribute to diabetes, aging, nerve damage, atherosclerosis, and deteriorations of the organ. Fasting with a healthy diet is a method for eliminating AGE from the cell tissue effectively.

If you do purified water quickly for more than a few days, the body runs out of carbohydrates to burn energy, triggering ketosis. In this situation, the body has to burn fat, and the fat storest chemicals and toxins from the atmosphere and foods we eat are retained in the body.

Médical reasons for fasting

The patient needs fast before the surgery to avoid complications when the body is trying to digest food during anesthesia. Other medical procedures for measuring cholesterol, blood sugar, and various laboratory tests are also needed to ensure accurate results.

Fasting to cure diseases,

Arthritis, lupus, skin conditions such as eczema and psoriasis have been removed by fasting to treat disease. Additionally, diseases of the digestive tract, such as colitis ulcer and Crohn's disease, were treated by distilled fasts. Also, low blood pressure was treated with fasting successfully.

The proceedings of the National Academy of Sciences and The Journal of Nutrition report studies showing that mice quickly had better insulin control, neuronal resistance, and several other health advantages than calorie-restricted mice when mice were forced to fast every other day. The mice receive twice the normal amount of food on the non-fasting day.

Fasting

Fasting Psychological advantages are used to cope with stress and depression through a lowering of chemical imbalances in the body. Many people should not be fast, including: pregnant women;

- ANICUS with any kind of malnutrition;
- people with heart problems;
- people with hepatic or renal failure.

Longevity fasting

Different studies demonstrate that animals live longer when feeding fewer calories.

In animals ranging from lizards to primates, their lifespans were extended when subjected to alternating periods of intense calorie-restricted diets and fasting. By comparison, the calorie-rich diets shorten human lives.

Live healthily and live longer with intermittent fasting, everyday workout, 8 to 10 glasses of distilled water a day, and a lot of fresh fruits and veggies.

Physical benefits of intermittent fasting

Many intermittent fasting benefits have been found by researchers who need to restrict caloric intake for some reason. Intermittent fasting is depicted as not eating for around fifteen hours. With this technique, many characteristics of the body can be improved. The official inquiry isn't whether fasting can support you, however, how it will help you and how frequently you ought to do it.

This style of fasting has been appeared to lower circulatory strain and increment HDL levels. It can extraordinarily help with overseeing diabetes, and it will enable you to get more fit too. These impacts sound quite tremendous and can be accomplished with this kind of fasting. Concentrates that have been done on several different species of creatures demonstrate that limiting caloric admission builds their lives by as much as 30 percent.

Concentrates on people demonstrate that it decreases pulse, glucose, and insulin affectability. With these tests, it makes sense that fasting, whenever accomplished for an extended period, will expand a human's life. Similar outcomes can be achieved by cutting your calories by 30 percent always. However, this has been appeared to cause wretchedness and fractiousness. Fasting is an answer that has been displayed in the spot of essentially cutting calories, and it has the benefits without the gloom or peevishness.

Intermittent fasting works by eating sustenance each other day. When that you do gobble, you will finish up eating twice as much food as you regularly would. You are as yet getting a similar measure of calories, yet you get the majority of the benefits too. It will lower stress levels and improve your general wellbeing levels. This kind of fasting is an incredible method to show signs of improving physical condition, to carry on with a more extended life, and to feel better always.

The Wonderful Benefits of Intermittent Fasting

The example of eating called "Intermittent Fasting" as a rule implies one fast for a timeframe and feeds for a deadline. Many pick a 24-hour cycle of fasting; at that point, eat well the following day and proceed with this procedure as a way of life change.

Research has been done on creatures to discover the advantages of this kind of fasting, and you will be glad to realize it indeed can be useful to your wellbeing!

Intermittent fasting can add 40%-56% more years to your life! That in itself is reason enough to do it. Anyway, different advantages incorporate bodyweight decrease and fat oxidation.

When you were quick, your body is compelled to search for fuel along these lines expelling matured and harmed cells simultaneously. This kind of purges the assemblage of annoying and undesirable things and helps the weight reduction and advantages of the significant nourishment decisions be expanded and progressively gainful to your body.

Rodents have been appeared to have a long haul and improved survival after heart disappointment after being on an IF eating plan, as well. Specialists are likewise saying that it may help age-related deficiencies in intellectual capacity, as well, with the goal that reveals to me that it may help avoid Alzheimer's Disease and different sorts of Dementia!

Your danger of coronary illness and other heart sicknesses may likewise be diminished when you begin a solid intermittent fasting routine. Your hazard for other interminable diseases and ailments will similarly doubtlessly be decreased.

A more beneficial you can start with intermittent fasting and reliable sustenance decisions! Keep carbs to 50-100 grams every day. Numerous ladies eat between 1200-1500 calories for each day, and when constraining their carbs, they are as yet shedding pounds. Men can deal with up to 2000 calories for each day. Less is ideal, and you have to determine caloric admission dependent on your action, for example, buckling down and working out.

Drink loads of liquids, particularly water, and exercise in the nights if conceivable. This will help with those late-night cravings.

Once you begin eating and drinking more beneficial, your body won't need to such an extent (assuming any) shoddy nourishment, so settling on reliable sustenance decisions will necessarily get more uncomplicated and more straightforward as you advance in the intermittent fasting schedule.

Substitute Day Fasting or ADF implies long rotating stretches of eating and not eating any sustenance, yet there is likewise intermittent fasting called Modified Fasting, where you devour about 20% of your typical calories one day and afterward eat ordinarily (yet sound) the following day. This is frequently progressively achievable for individuals since they feel less denied when they can, at any rate, eat something every day, despite everything it has the vast majority of the advantages of the ADF routine.

Whatever you do, ensure you tell your therapeutic services proficient of your arrangements so the person in question knows and can work with you to achieve your objectives. If you need to get in shape, lose fat, and feel much improved, at that point intermittent fasting may be the response for you!

Intermittent Fasting and Bodybuilding: How to Make It Work for You

Is it only a fleeting sensation, or is it digging in for the long haul? Intermittent fasting appears to have appeared suddenly in a previous couple of months. Intermittent fasting, which is an entirely extravagant (now and again off-putting) state for what is essentially two windows - a window when to eat and a window when not to eat.

Intermittent fasting and lifting weights can work for you if you will probably construct muscle and to get slender, and here are three reasons why.

1. Ongoing examinations have demonstrated that it is an established truth all out macros and the aggregate sum of every day calories that represent muscle development and not the measure of meals and the planning of them. Essentially this is stating that as long as you get the required standard of calories in the 24 hours, it doesn't make a difference when you get them. So as long as you understand you required a measure of calories (an overflow of your TDEE is needed for the mix with a dynamic preparing schedule) in your eating window, you will pick up muscle.

2. One feature of intermittent fasting weight training that individuals whine about is the measure of sustenance and calories that should be expended inside the eaten window. Even though you in all probability should alter if you are right now eating 6-8 light meals daily, over two or three weeks, your stomach will conform to eating more substantial meals. I thought that it was tough to eat large meals in the first place; however, within a week or so, I balanced, and now I have no issues securing large measures of sustenance in one sitting. Take as much time as is required with the adjustment period and don't hope to have the capacity to switch overnight.

3. Keep in mind, such as everything else, intermittent fasting isn't an exact science, and if you have to expand our eating window from state an eight-hour eating window to a nine-hour window to suit your total calories and dinner necessities, that is fine feel free to do as such. Like any program, it's imperative to discover what works for you. Intermittent fasting, weight training, and building muscle can cooperate, and its excellence is if you locate that sweet recognize that works for you-you'll get the advantages of intermittent fasting while at the same time keeping up or assembling your constitution to a lifting weights level.

Weight reduction: Intermittent Fasting

The standard eating regimens where you cut your calorie admission amid the whole eating routine, either by reducing the carbs or fats, are gradually ending up less well known. Imagine a scenario in which you can eat your preferred sustenance and still lose the muscle to fat ratio.

The Intermittent Fasting diet speaks to an example of eating that switches back and forth between time of not eating (fasting) and a time of eating (additionally called a sustaining window). The fasting stage is a timeframe where no calories are expended (no one but water can be devoured or relying upon the methodology some thick calorie beverages like espresso). The nourishing window is the point at which you devour entire sustenance. On a more extended term, this sort of eating will make calorie shortfall (eating fewer calories than your body consumes).

As indicated by various examinations, there are multiple advantages to Intermittent Fasting. Weight reduction is the greatest one of them. Amid the fast, muscle versus fat is utilized as an energy source rather than put away glycogen. Amid the quick HGH (Human growth hormone which jam bulk and enables consume to fat) is discharged in the circulatory system, and furthermore, Insulin levels are diminished, which implies that your body will store less fat.

There are a couple of ways to deal with Intermittent Fasting:

· Sixteen hours fast, trailed by an 8-hour nourishing window (Lean gains diet).
· Twenty hours fast, trailed by a 4-hour bolstering window.
· 24-hour fasts a couple of times each week.

Furthermore, there is additionally the Warrior Diet, where you can break the fasting time frame by eating little portions of vegetables or products of the soil dosages of protein.

A genuine case of the Intermittent Fasting diet is the Lean gains diet where you adjust between 16 hours fast and an 8 hour bolstering period:

· The fast can start at 8 p.m. Furthermore, last till noon a few days ago.

Usually, people are dynamic toward the beginning of the day, either by working or doing their morning exercise.

· Noon first and biggest feast - half of the absolute calories

· 4 p.m. second feast - 25% of the absolute calories

· 7-8 p.m. last feast - 25% of the absolute calories

Why You Should Try Intermittent Fasting

Intermittent fasting is a dubious weight reduction system since it includes not eating sustenance for an all-inclusive timeframe. Numerous individuals have the idea that not eating will hinder your digestion and send your body into starvation mode, yet it turns out this isn't valid in any way. The human body was intended to go significant lots of time without eating, so intermittent fasting is a personal practice. Maybe that is the reason it is so viable.

If you might want to get in shape, however, would prefer not to surrender specific sustenance or would prefer not to share in vivacious exercise, intermittent fasting is presumably your best alternative. Fasting will enable you to shed pounds immediately, regardless of whether you don't eat very sound or activity, although that would extraordinarily upgrade your outcomes. This procedure doesn't expect you to bring down the measure of calories you devour. It just takes a tad of order to start with.

If you don't care for fasting, maybe the benefits will persuade you out it an attempt in any case. Intermittent fasting has numerous benefits that will extraordinarily increase a fantastic nature. A portion of the benefits include:

· Rapid fat misfortune

· Lowered pulse and cholesterol

· Increase in vitality, particularly in the mornings

· Enhanced memory and psychological capacity

These are only a couple of the numerous benefits that fasting can offer you. If you necessarily need to be a more advantageous or potentially more joyful individual, it would be of your best enthusiasm to start an intermittent fasting schedule. Taking everything into account, in what manner may you start?

There are several different ways one can start fasting. One technique, the one I like, is everyday fasting. This includes eating your sustenance for the day inside a timeframe of 6 to 8 hours. This would mean you quick for 16 to 18 hours consistently. The most straightforward approach to do this is to skip breakfast in the mornings. You will profit enormously from this. Considerably more significant benefits will be experienced when you can stretch the time spent fasting. For instance, quick for 20 hours and eat for 4. Make sense of what works best for you.

Another technique that likewise functions admirably is week by week fasting. This would include a time of fasting that lasts between 24 and 36 hours. Along these lines, for instance, you would eat as you regularly accomplish for six days of the week; at that point, one day you would not eat any nourishment whatsoever. Drink a lot of water amid when you are not eating. Week after week, fasting is additionally successful, however not as powerful as daily fasting I have found. I urge you to find out more and start to fuse one of these procedures into your life.

Helpful Low Carb Intermittent Fasting

When you are thinking about low carb intermittent fasting, you will need to make a point to peruse the whole section.

Intermittent fasting implies fasting for a decided measure of time (numerous individuals quick 24 hours at that point eat healthy the following 24 hours, etc.). This means your body needs to search around for sustenance (fuel), and in the process, disposes of awful matured or harmed cells and other waste that has developed in your body.

Consolidate the two of these for "Low Carb Intermittent Fasting," and you'll have a triumphant blend to getting in shape and feeling extraordinary!

When you are fasting, you can, in any case, have low carb and low-calorie beverages, for example, water, and dark espresso, however, you ought not to eat foods for 24 hours. You can eat healthy the next day. However, you should, in any case, keep watch on your carbohydrate admission. Peruse marks and research foods to realize you are settling on the best choices for your body and your wellbeing.

"Live," or fresh foods are always incredible choices. Keep in mind garbage in methods garbage out, and healthy decisions mean a more advantageous lifestyle. This is a lifestyle change and ought to be a steady method for eating for you (at any rate the low carbs). You need to try to settle on astute sustenance and drink choices!

Join low carb intermittent fasting alongside exercise, and you'll be fit as a fiddle before you know it and will feel incredible.

Intermittent fasting diminishes fat oxidation and may lessen bodyweight. Practicing will speed the procedure along and will enable you to dispose of overweight skin and get conditioned.

Intermittent fasting that has been led on creatures demonstrate a life expectancy increment of 40% or more. That is stunning! This shows how much eating healthy and purifying your body can profit, not just your framework, and help you get thinner, yet it can likewise expand your days on this planet.

Low carb nourishment choices are vegetables. You can necessarily eat the same number of the plant as you need. Meats and fish are great supper choices. For lunch, you could make a serving of mixed greens with a bubbled egg, onion, and a dash of cheddar. Watch the carbs in the dressing, however.

For whatever period that you are resolved to settle on healthy lifestyle choices, your craving for sugars and carbs will no doubt be no more. That craving will be diminished! You'll never again need greasy, sweet foods, when you begin settling on the choice to eat healthy, low carb foods.

Drink bunches of water, as well. Different refreshments that are great are dark espresso and green tea; however, don't try too hard on the caffeine. What's more, recollect before beginning any eating regimen plan or exercise schedule, dependably check with your therapeutic services proficient! You need to ensure you remain healthy while getting more advantageous!

Chapter Two:
Five MOST Silly Reasons Women Die

Men don't look after themselves. They are not eating right. We are not eating right. They're pushing too hard. They won't tell anyone if something's wrong until they're on the door of death. We maintain alarming signs and symptoms. You don't seem to mind if you die young and leave your family without fathers or husbands. It's true too often, but we guys also have some impressive features. In caring and defending our loved ones, we are courageous, strong, trustworthy, and passionate. Nonetheless, we still die off quicker. So as a doctor, I have spent a large part of my working time working around the average man's love of avoiding health care.

We inspire our children to participate in every aspect of their lives, in schools, in sports, and in business. The high-level boss, the prosecutor, the doctor, is also considered to be a "catch" by both sexes. How many people do admire someone else who has chosen a low/low pay career because he wants to be "personal?" And what dad would his daughter like to marry a grocer rather than a high-earning investor?

Nevertheless, the grocery worker could have less work stress and more involvement in the lives of his wife and children. Helping us to live longer and healthier starts with the awareness of our competitive nature, and I'd point to two excellent books by Warren Farrell, Ph.D.: Why are people the way they are and the illusion of man's power.

So what does the list of dumb reasons to die take? Each member of this list has two qualities: either of disease kills a large number of people in spite of proper screening and prevention or...
It is a very rare cause of death, but it is very clear and easy to prevent.

ı would probably remember a lot of people, famous, family or friends, who died from one of these five causes. We'll each look separately, but here's first my shortlist of Men die for silly bad reasons:

1. Heart attack or stroke is dying because treatable risk factors have been underestimated.

2. Dying of Colon Cancer for fear that anything would stick there.

3. Prostate Cancer death because you have never had a blood test.

4. Dying of Malignant Melanoma because it was a symbol of beauty, you thought.

5. Apnea's death from sleep when snoring is snoring.

Lung cancer is not identified as one of the dumb causes of men's death, as the vast majority of men are conscious that smoking is likely to cause it. You have implicitly acknowledged this threat by smoking, while risk-free, in exchange for any psychological benefits or because of an unmistakable dependence.

1. Silly Reason #1: The Big One killer of this country is the one we call THE BIG ONE, a cardio-vascular case in the medical business. They build widows and caregivers. These are almost always the product of the so-called arterial hardening, a very complex process called the Atherosclerotic Arterial Disease.

Men usually experience hardening of the arteries faster than women. Much of this was due to the obvious protective effects of the female hormone, estrogen since the female arteries begin to catch up to men only after menopause. There are a variety of well-known risk factors associated with heart attacks that every man over the age of 30 and even younger men with a family history of heart attack or stroke should tackle.

The major risk factors for cardiovascular diseases (CV). The major risk factor is a "yes" answer to this question:

Has this person hardened arteries already? Those who have already had a stroke or heart attack are more likely to have one in the future. Patients with their coronary arteries hardening (feeding the heart) or their carotid arteries (feeding the brain) are next in line.

2. The second-largest risk factor for THE BIG ONE lies in the family of heart diseases or stroke among brothers, sisters, parents, and children and, to a lesser degree, among grandparents and aunts and uncles linked to blood. No matter if a man has good cholesterol or blood pressure and has two brothers who died from a heart attack, he's a walking time bomb before tests show otherwise.

3. Elevated Cholesterol Serum! Everyone knows this evil substance in the country. It's on tv, in our fitness magazines-about everywhere people share their thoughts, and some of the most popular food and diet marketing strategies in history have been fuelled. And this is false! And it is wrong! Most people with a heart attack or stroke have normal cholesterol levels. Nonetheless, most of these patients would probably have done much better if they had reduced the amount of cholesterol.

4. Total cholesterol of the patient is highest if below 200. Most importantly, LDL should be less than 130 (bad cholesterol). In men, HDL (good cholesterol) should be higher than 40 and for women higher than 50. The number of triglycerides should be lower than 150. The inability to control high cholesterol by the most efficient therapeutic procedure will contribute significantly to the death of another healthy human being. 4. High blood pressure, also known as high blood pressure. While it is necessary to maintain blood flowing through the pipes, blood pressure may be too high for long-term wear on these pipes. Coronary arteries, the little arteries that support the heart itself, never stop and pause— the heart works 24 hours a day, seven days a week. In this system, higher blood

pressure can cause atherosclerotic changes to these arteries, which results in heart attack and death.

5. Tobacco. Smoking. Realize that one regular cigarette smoking risk of a heart attack is exactly the same as smoking a pack per day. It doesn't help much to cut down. You must stop. You must stop. This is different from the risk that smoking adds to lung cancer, which reduces your chances of this disease significantly. Heart attack and stroke are less about how much in one day you smoke and more about smoking.

6. In modern medicine, diabetes is not redefined as a disease that one has or does not, but rather as a late complication of a more complex, subtle, and invisible phase, called insulin resistance. Proper diabetic screening requires not merely a quick glucose test but also an assessment of potential insulin resistance, first by checking to fast and then blood insulin levels post-breakfast.

7. The ultimate major risk factor is the male sex itself. We can't do much about this one.

Other emerging risk factors are more widely understood and regulated. These include homocysteine, lipoprotein A, fibrinogen level, very responsive C reactive protein, plasminogen activator inhibitor, apoprotein-E genotype, interleukin-6, and TNF as well as my currently favored LDL and HDL gel electrophoresis.

Please understand, no diet or exercise can prevent a man from having a heart attack or a stroke if the above tests and associated treatments are omitted.

Colonic cancer is one of the stupidest cancers on the planet and should no longer have any chance to kill the American average man or woman. Like lung cancer, colon cancer is one of the stupidest cancers on the earth. This starts as a slow-growing, low-grade, and visible tumor and takes years to develop into a murderer who spreads and murders you everywhere. The only trick it uses is stubbornness. It hides in a place people hate to look.

Modern tortoise and hare: colon cancer tortoise plays on patiently while we are dumb. We put off a colonoscopy, which is probably painful if we can't face it or refuse to pay for it. Dumb! Dumb!

Silly Reason #3: Sorry, No End Again Prostate cancer doesn't develop as slowly as easily curable early stages, but is easily taken up in the majority of patients by routine testing in a curable form. Make sure every year you get the PSA blood test. That alone could save hundreds of thousands of lives every year. Every year after age 40, it is better to have the traditional "finger wave" (rectoral exam) and the PSA test, but when I can only choose one, the blood test is the most sensitive screening process.

Following cancer, malignant melanoma, is similarly true for men and women as well, which uses a killing technique that is exactly the opposite of the tortoise and hare method of more laid-back colon cancer. The following cancer is malignant melanoma. Hides melanoma in the plain. Like colon cancer, it flies out of hell like a bat. It is a black spot that is easily discovered (sometimes ironically called a' beauty sign'), which can be anticipated and easily removed if it is discovered in time. All that is required is to look in the mirror or watch each other's mutual back.

Dumb Reason #5: Dangerous sleep The end of my shortlist of top five silly reasons is a common problem of sleep called obstructive sleep apnea— deadly snoring. About 6% of all American men have this sleep disorder, but few die as a result. Sleep apnea ("sleep no respiration") leads to a mechanical air-off when the muscles in the neck slurry during deep sleep. The resulting intermittent low levels of oxygen cause lung damage for a long time. Over the years, this damage leads to heart failure and death. Apart from snoring, a sleepy life, which is chronically exhausted, is normal because these patients ' brains will not allow you to stay in a deep sleep for over a minute. The imminent suffocation allows the individual to return to a much lighter sleep to keep the airway open. Even if patients sleep ten hours a night, they often wake up exhausted and fall asleep often and quickly throughout the day.

Diet Plans For Women Of All Ages

We all want to live healthy and young for as long as possible. For years, scientists have been working to find a way to extend our lives.

They found that the reduction in calories—a dramatic reduction in calories consumed over long periods—can extend the lives of many animals, and also probably the lives of men and women. Sadly, the restriction of calories is very complicated and requires a total commitment to the lifestyle.

It also has severe side effects. It can contribute to eating disorders, depression, and hormones so that men look more like women, and when they practice calory restriction, they become masculine.

Nevertheless, recent experiments with another method of eating alteration have led to life extension advantages for animals: intermittent fasting. Rats fed 24 hours, fasted 24 hours, live longer than regularly fed rats, even though in the food, they eat almost as many calories. And there are many benefits of intermittent fasting over calorie limits. The main one is that it is faster, but it has also not been linked to depression, dietary problems, or hormonal changes.

When a person prepares for intermittent fasting, his energy level will not be impaired—our ancestors would never have survived if they had three square meals a day to work—and even on fasting days, they can do their normal activities.

So if you want an anti-aging approach that is easy to use and does not have many side effects, try intermittent fasting.

The Wonderful Benefits of Intermittent Fasting

The eating pattern called "intermittent fasting" usually means that you fast for a certain time and eat for a certain period of time. Most choose a 24-hour fasting process, then eat healthy the next day, and keep on improving their way of life.

Animals are studied to find the benefits of this form of raping, and you will be glad to know that it can really improve your wellbeing!

Intermittent fasting will add 40 -56% more years to your life! That alone is sufficient reason to do so. Certain advantages include decreased body weight and fat oxidation.

If you quickly scavenge your body for fuel, removing old and damaged cells. It cleanses the body of unnecessary and unused stuff and helps to improve the weight loss and benefits of good food decisions and to support the health.

Rat's long-term and enhanced survival were demonstrated after heart failure, also in the sense of an IF food plan. Experts also suggest that it may improve age-related cognitive function problems too, which can help to prevent Alzheimer's and other forms of dementia!

You may also decrease the risk of heart disease and other heartaches by beginning a regular, irregular, rapid regimen. The risk will most probably also be may for other chronic disorders and diseases.

You can start healthier with intermittent fasting and healthy food choices! Hold 50-100 grams of carbs per day. Many women eat between 1200 and 1500 calories daily and still lose weight when limiting their carbs. Up to 2000, calories can be handled per day by men. Of example, less is healthier, and caloric intake must be determined based on your activities such as hard work and exercise.

Drink lots of fluids, especially water, and, where possible, exercise at night. It helps with those cravings late at night.

When you begin eating and drinking responsibly, your body won't want as much (if any) junk food, so it'll be easier to make healthy food choices as you go through intermittent fasting.

Alternate day fasts or ADF means alternate fasting days and no food, but an intermittent fast is also known as adjusted fasts, where you consume about 20% of your usual calories one day and then eat regular (but healthy) the next day. This is often more realistic as people feel less fortunate if they can at least eat something every day and still have most of the advantages of the ADF system.

Make sure you tell the health care provider what you want to do so that he or she is aware of your intentions and can work with you to reach your goals. If you want to lose weight, lose fat, and feel better, intermittent quacking maybe your response!

Intermittent Fasting, What Is It and Is It For You?

There is a new child in the city called Intermittent Fasting, and a lot of scientific knowledge about it has good things to say.

At least six models are created by as many fans and several doctors, each of them with a twist when you eat and don't and how much. The results vary from the reduction of fat and weight to better memory and long-term disease prevention.

Let's begin with a little science on fasting physiology.

The body goes into a digestive mode when we eat. Insulin increases because the absorption of this meal creates blood sugar. It will last from 3 to 5 hours. You are in post-absorption mode once you are fed, and food is digested. It ensures the nutrients are stored and consumed. Insulin has gone down, back to normal. You're in fasting mode now. The longer you stay here, the more likely it is that the body will eat stored fat. Yet spend too much time here, and the body consumes muscle and lower metabolism as a way to maintain energy stores.

The key is quick enough, and how long is heatedly debated to burn stored fat and the advantages of calorie restriction without the mentioned downsides.

The easiest of these strategies is that food is within an 8-hour window—eight hours and 16 easily doesn't matter. It might look like eight meals, skipping breakfast and eating once more.

Confusion is just in place. Isn't breakfast missing terribly for you?

For some, it's going to be. This isn't the plan for you if you're hypoglycemic.

For others, the body adapts, you will not die, and the effects of traditional diets will blast from the windows in people who want to lose weight.

Why is this mostly because it is simpler than how much or what you consume to restrict eating times.

There are other plans, Krista Varady's Every Other Day Diet, a scientist who is well-researched and successful. You eat the way it sounds, you fast or feast every other day. One interesting finding from Krista's study is that most people do not eat enough during the feast day to avoid weight loss.

Martin Berkhan was called IF and had a number of options to pursue.

Precision Nutrition's John Berardi is a qualified dietitian in his words. In other words, he checks diets and fitness programs. He has the best free IF weight loss and wellbeing app. Here you can pick it up. He has checked almost every variation with which you can come up. Since it is still important to work out, he discusses when he needs to work out quickly.

It should be noted that his final word, whether it works for weight loss and whether it is healthy or not, is that many programs work if the person is appropriate and sticks to that. It's only one way.

There are extreme versions of this definition in which you eat 500 calories one day and then the next day, then immediately for two days, and so on. Even as a launchpad, I'm never a fan of extremes. If it sounds like an idea or you just want to try and see how you feel, and if you lose weight, start by shortening the hours you'll eat on the day you eat as I mentioned in the first scenario.

Apart from smaller thighs, what else is good?

Intermittent fasting is in the class of calorie limits that have been well-researched by science to maximize lifetime.

Chapter Three:
The Easiest Diet is - Eat Stop Eat

Eat Stop Eat is a fasting diet intermittently. What is intermittent quicking? It is when you usually eat for a period of time and then quickly for a period of time.

Eat Stop Eat takes a simple dietary approach. There is no calorie count or another trick where the food you eat and drink must be noted. This diet plan is based on the idea that the more restrictive the diet, the more likely that you will fail. It refers to many men. Many people don't have the ability to write down what they eat at any exact time.

As Eat Stop Eat reiterates, the basic principle of weight loss produces a calorie deficit. Where calories come from, it does not matter, as long as you keep them below the amount you need to use to lose weight. You can essentially eat anything you want, as long as you remain within a certain amount.

Eating Stop Eat gives rise to the misconception that not eating every couple of hours can lead to muscle loss. This should be a given, as the typical eating style was only eaten three times a day. Although muscle growth depends heavily on protein, skipping one or two meals does not lead to muscle loss.

Eat Stop Eat recently became one of the internet's best-selling diets. It's no surprise with such a relaxed approach to eating. We even have different sections for both men and women. Whether you are young or old, this diet plan might be the right diet for you.

~!@#$%$@$$! @#$%$

For me, Eat Stop Eat is the best diet for fat loss. Designed by Brad Pilon, a licensed nutritionist focuses on intermittent fasting, moderate weight-training for building lean muscle mass, increasing your natural metabolism, and your daily physical activity. Eat Stop Eat is NOT a fading diet, nor a fast loss of weight. This promotes positive lifestyle improvements and life-long behaviors.

Why use the best diet?

Plain. Simple. The simplest diet to start, manage, and see observable results is the one with which you can confirm most easily. Although all dieting programs should work for the first several weeks, you will lose interest in staying with them if complex methods are used to calculate quantities, boring newspaper research, or monitoring or restrictive food choices. A fat loss program that focuses on improving your food choices, regularly exercising, drinking more water, and rest is a simple diet to sustain... Because it focuses on making positive changes to your lifestyle.

What is intermittent fasting, and why is it good?

Intermittent rapidity is a technique to achieve a fat loss calorie deficit. It's never finished for 24 hours. It's never done in a row for two days. You snack every day with Snack Stop Food. Some people quickly start after dinner, then don't eat before the next day's evening meal. You NEVER go a day without feeding, yet you will lose fat by generating an average weekly calorie deficit. Contrary to what you read in pop fitness literature, because this is not an extended hunger technique, you won't lose muscle. It is a safe and sensitive way to reduce your caloric consumption.

The best plan for fat loss is positive. A simple diet results in nutrition and resilience. Most weight loss programs in less than 30 days guarantee dramatic declines in pounds. Nonetheless, the best weight loss plans are only 1-2 lbs. Every week. It may not seem important when you look at it stretched over 12 months... it will then open your eyes. I found this to be the best diet for women due to the simplicity of eating stop and its progressive approach to fat loss.

Description Nothing is required to indulge in starvation-like diets, complex food schedules, extreme exercise habits, expensive drugs, or unsafe pills. Remember that the simplest diet is without a lot of scattered work or complex tasks. You are losing fat healthily and progressively if you sense a calorie deficit by making better food choices, participate in daily exercises of a moderate weight training and exercise 30-40 minutes per day instead of watching television and e-mails. Eat Stop Eat is a fast and worthwhile diet plan.

Ways to Increase Growth Hormone

Growth Hormone (also known as GH) was given a lot of attention recently, as a number of professional athletes and celebrities were speculated to use the hormone, and some were handed over purple. And why anybody would ever like to take growth hormone?

Research has shown that injections of growth hormones will increase the magnitude and decrease the mass of fat! Increases in lean mass are related to an increase in metabolism so that more calories are consumed. A drop in fat mass doesn't have to be clarified why everyone would be involved in this! Hollywood reports also say that GH injections will make your skin look younger. In short, this substance is the proverbial root of young people.

Natural growth hormone levels start to decline rapidly in both men and women at the end of the 20s. The decline is thought to be GH, partially, which makes us look and feel older as we age.

Those who have the financial resources and a doctor who is prepared to prescribe GH can use GH to stay young. Many professional athletes and bodybuilders may turn to the black market to find GH, but this is not a wise idea because it is illegal, and its consistency and purity can not be verified. As amazing as the growth hormone sounds, a prescription and the doctor will check to confirm that you need it. And as far as I know, doctors don't just send GH prescriptions to everyone who comes to work, who needs them to restore their bodies and looks in their 20's.

We have discussed up to now one way to increase growth hormone by using it as a medicine, but there are two easier and cheaper ways to increase growth hormones that do not need a doctor or a prescription: intense workout and fasting!

Indeed, you read correctly, and it has been shown that short-time fasting dramatically increases the growth hormone levels by as much as six times! This rise is even greater than the amounts injected into muscle mass increases by researchers.

Because of its supposed capacity to slow down the aging process, growth hormone draws much interest and allows people to look younger. Short-term intermittent fasting and intensive exercises are very effective ways of increasing growth hormone levels safely and regularly.

Health Benefits Of Fasting From Time To Time

Intermittent fasting is a dietary schedule that alternates between normal eating and fasting times. There are numerous intermittent fasting programs to choose from, and the cycles between the diet and the program can vary. Another example is the 5:2 diet, which includes five days of normal eating and then 1/4 of your recommended daily calorie allowance on the two remaining days. Most easily on two straight days, and some tend to do so on separate days, such as a Monday and a Thursday.

There are many good reasons for fasting intermittently. Advantages of fasting regularly Many people see this food plan as part of a weight reduction strategy. Rushing sometimes will help increase your sensitivity to insulin, which generally leads to a more noticeable weight loss. This is because the higher the body's response to insulin, the more you lose fat and gain muscle. The sensitivity of insulin is higher after 8-10 hours and after exercise. Therefore, proponents of this diet, most of the time, advocate exercise even in fasting to lose more weight. It may also allow you to reduce triglyceride and LDL levels once or twice a week. Intermittent fasting can also improve the secretion of growth hormone with countless health benefits, particularly its ability to resist cortisol effects such as fat storage in the belly. The quick is also related to things like increased longevity and decreased risk of developing heart problems, which is close to other kinds of caloric restrictions.

Why can't quick every now and then?

Although this dietary approach is effective and beneficial, it can cause unwanted effects for individual groups. Those who recover from surgery are not expected to rapidly. You should not do this too if you feel ill or have a fever. Diabetic patients, particularly insulin patients, and maintainers, need to talk to their doctor before fasting intermittently. In addition, babies, as well as the women who are pregnant or breastfeeding, should not use this diet.

Do I have side effects?

Hunger is one of the anticipated side effects of swiftness, especially when you start. You will gradually feel less hunger, even if you eat less often.

In addition, intermittent fasting is not to be seen as a diet, but as a natural way of life. This approach does not extend to everyone, but it is definitely a successful way to lose weight and stay healthy.

What Are the Best Ways to Eat Healthy at Work?

The best way to get used to lunch every day is to do it the previous night. Mornings can be noisy. Imagine this: the alarm clothes you sleep, and your son loses his school bus. There's very little hope that in this situation you will prepare your lunch. These morning monkey wrinkles are quite common for women with careers and families. A great time saver I use is to cook enough food and prepare it for the next day's lunch.

I recommend that my patients eat as healthy as possible six days a week and have a cheat day to satisfy cravings and stresses, to reset hormones, and to fire you throughout the week. If you can have junk food, it will lose its appeal whenever you want. A slice of cheesecake is much more satisfying if you have to wait until Saturday to eat it. Each meal should be served a protein source during the six days of our "healthy" diet, including poultry, turkey, grass-fed beef, tuna and ovaries, a source of carbohydrates like quinoa, bean or brown rice (small quantities) and plenty of green vegetables including cakes and spinach. One good way to make your greens delicious is to add a sparkling black pepper and sea salt to the grass-fed butter.

There are two ways to avoid snacking the dreaded delicacies: eat until every meal is satiated and not useful. There is less temptation to snack between meals if you are full after meals. Therefore, if there are no Oreos in the cabinet next to your desk, you are less in danger of falling into temptation. I recommend snack raw almonds or cashews, kale chips, Greek yogurt, whey powder protein, hummus, and sticks.

If you want to get clean, you must have tunnel vision. We're always being bombarded by fast-food ads, advertising for all that you want buffets, and even colleagues who feel like they need to make sarcastic remarks or try to convince you of that by living a healthy lifestyle. When I make my health a priority, my coworkers feel uncomfortable or insulted, then they have issues with which to deal, not me, but people who skip lunch tend to eat junk food or overeat at dinner. My thumb rule is not to save lunch.

I'd rather eat with others to break up the day's monotony. If I have to improve productivity or stay at work, I eat at my office. It's all about choice.

The best way to get back on track after a rough week is to get back straight on the horse. Over a bad week, you can't beat yourself. This is a daily battle.

Chapter Four:
How to Increase HGH – Naturally

It's no secret that we don't get our ancestors ' education. We choose our meat from a supermarket cooler, but not from long, successful hunting expeditions. Few of us understand how hard it is to grow enough fruits and vegetables to feed our families.

In the past, fasting was a way of life, simply because food "caught as catch" was literally. We now realize that this system has advantages.

Our body enters a cycle of the breakdown of tissue (called "catabolic"), when we fly, allowing the body to remove, harm, and replace it with stronger cells.

They were much slimmer, body fat that today would be the envy of the elite. It was usually less than 10% for men and 10-20% for women. Recent research suggests that at least part of this old lifestyle can be useful to recreate.

It ensures that the intermittent fasting and high-intensity, short-term workouts will keep us safer and healthier.

But the best part is here: we all know about the commercial got from HGH (Human Growth Hormone). Now some recent studies have shown the intriguing possibility that irregular rapidity combined with exercise in high intensity in brief blasts actually enhances HGH in the body.

The Intermountain Medical Center Heart Institute in Murray and Utah (near Salt Lake City), as well as the British Journal of Sports Medicine, published results.

The study in Utah focussed on the impact of fasting and found that men were able to increase their HGH by 2000% and women by 1300%.

The British research dealt with the use of lactic acid, of course. It is well understood that an accumulation of lactic acid will cause the production of HGH, but human beings cannot withstand the physical discomfort caused by the production of enough lactic acid.

But researchers are now connecting data from these two previously unrelated studies and coming to a startling conclusion: a controlled rapid regime, combined with high-intensity aerobic exercises, will spontaneously increase human growth hormone in the body.

Although most doctors say that every workout is helpful, low-intensity exercise uses the body, whereas high-intensity workouts help healthy tissue repair.

While more research is coming, the proof so far is that brief bursts of exercise of high intensity are the most banging of all.

Easily Reduce Your Fat Percentage

If you want a tighter body, your eyes are excess fat. You want this fat level to be that.

This is the explanation for many people to eat less and to significantly reduce the number of calories. In theory, this is a good way to lose fat. But whether that benefits you in the long term as well?
In this chapter, we share a few simple ways of reducing the fat content and ensuring that it stays away.

How can you reduce your fat?
Do you want a good way to get rid of your extra pounds? The fat on your belly is not a proud part of your body. That is reason you want to say farewell. To get rid of that excess fat, you need to do some different things. Make a conscious effort of eating healthier and better consider this part of your everyday life. You're going to lose your fat.

Be Patience

You have to take the time to remove your fat percentage. All can lose their fat percentage at a different pace. Stop aggressive crash diets, in which too few calories are consumed, and you are totally starving. Reducing your fat percentage requires a healthy diet and takes time.

Don't stand on the scales every day, so take advantage of the small body shifts. Step by step changes the way you eat a number of things. This makes it easy to succeed in the long run. You will then be able to reduce the fat percentage.

Alternative carbohydrates

Everyone doesn't need to modify your carbohydrates, but it can help lower your fat percentage. Many days you eat lots of carbohydrates, and some days, you eat small carbohydrates, which ensures the body automatically has a deficit of calories.

You eat a lot of carbohydrates before you undergo intensive training. And you don't need these calories if you don't practice. You eat less of it, too.

As you only get a lot of calories during your workouts, they have burned again instantly. This way of eating means that despite eating low calories, you will continue to exercise intensively.

Egg whites

Proteins are one of the essential substances to develop the muscles. Proteins are also important to reduce the percentage of fat. For your muscles, proteins are important building materials. Proteins ensure that your muscles are strengthened as you lose weight.

It is good to know that muscle tissue is more energy-efficient than fat. You always have enough strength by eating enough protein.

Another great benefit of protein-rich meals is that you have a sense of satiety. Adding this to your eating pattern will stop hunger. It means that you eat less and lose your fat percentage quickly.

Less calories

Many people decide to exercise a lot and eat more healthily if they want to lose a lot of weight. You just lose fat, though, if you reduce the amount of calories too. You always need less calories than your body needs. You know exactly how many calories you have to eat, you have to know what the calorie requirements are for your body.

The Harris and Benedict formula is a well-known formula to use. The great advantage of a low-calorie reduction is that you retain muscle mass during weight loss in this way. You can stop the uncomfortable sensation of hunger. It makes mental health much simpler.

Strength training and exercise

The second objective is to improve the muscles and, therefore, your energy consumption in addition to reducing your fat percentage. You eat fewer calories in conjunction with exercise every day.

It is best to use yoga as well as strength training to burn more calories. You can use a short, vigorous exercise for up to 15 minutes of interval training, with which you can consume extra calories. Then for hours, you don't have to use a treadmill or cross-trainer.

Eating Vegetable

Gastronomy One of the easiest things to reduce your weight is to eat more vegetables. The big advantage of vegetables is that they make you feel satiety, have good nutrients, and are low in calories.

Different fruit and vegetables provide a strong fiber source, which suppresses the feeling of hunger.

However, it is much more fun to suck on some fruit than to feel hungry.

Right Nutrients

Make sure you have fewer calories per day if you want to lower your fat percentage.

In order to maintain this way of eating and make it as fun as possible, you have to get healthy food. These are the foods that provide you with enough vitamins and minerals. Think of fruit and vegetables. Avoid a lot of refined sugar ingredients, including cookies and candy.

Beverages It is good to avoid calories from beverages while raising the fat percentage. If only a certain number of calories are required to be eaten per day, keep them from being concealed in your drink. However, these drinks don't give you a sense of satiety.

Drink

Drink a drink of low calories, such as tea, soda, or coffee. Do not bring your coffee or tea with sugar or milk.

One of the best ways to treat your body well is by drinking plenty of water. We all know it's good for our bodies, so we drink too little. To our bodies, this is not healthy.

Water is good for different body functions and can also help you reduce your fat percentage. Many people don't know a sense of hunger anymore but perceive it as a feeling of starvation. That's why drinking enough during the day is necessary.

Different studies have shown that you drink a glass of water before a meal if you consume less. Make sure every day you get between 1.5 and 2 liters of water. For athletes, the fluid you lose due to sweating should be replenished.

Learning When to Eat What to Maximize Muscle and Burn Fat

Protein type/protein timing

The aim is to consume the most ideal possible so that everyone who wants to maximize muscle development and reduce storage for excess calories as body fat will provide a constant stream of nutrients, and blood sugar levels always stay constant. Apart from eating high-quality, low-fat foods, one of the most effective ways to achieve this is to eat small, regular foods (every 2 to 3 hours). Successful bodybuilders know that they provide their muscles with a steady stream of nutrients while eating at least six evenly spaced meals the whole day long, which keeps their body in anabolic conditions (as a positive nitrogen balance).

Especially when it comes to protein consumption, it is very important to eat smaller, more frequent meals because proteins can not be stored in the body as carbohydrates can (carbohydrates can be stored in the liver as glycogen and used until days later if needed).

Because there is only a very small amount of amino acid within the bloodstream, full proteins should be consumed with all meals to maintain an anabolic (muscle building) environment. The sudden and high increase in amino acid levels in the blood causes the rate of protein synthesis to rise and protein breakdown to decrease.

The preservation of a proper nitrogen balance prevents the body from collapsing into its own tissue (catabolism) to receive nutrients that it requires (such as protein). Therefore, it is important to eat 5 to 6 protein-containing meals per day (each about every two to 3 hours) containing around 30-40 grams of protein, so that a positive nitrogen balance is maintained (which comes from the amino acid breakdown).

Large, evenly spread foods maintain a stable level of insulin, a need for good fat metabolism, and good growth. It is also easier to eat in the digestive system and more effective. Research has shown that consuming many smaller foods improves metabolic rates, burns more calories, and contributes to less body fat accumulation. The rate of protein digestion has significant effects on the body's protein balance. The combination of protein synthesis and the degradation of a protein determines muscle gain.

Protein is usually called "quick digestion" or "slow digestion." Nevertheless, successful bodybuilders need to take protein time one step more to maximize muscle syntheses. Protein timing also means eating the "best" protein at the right time. What does that mean? What does that mean?
Nutrition is a very individual problem. There will be no single diet for everyone.

While there are common strategies that work properly for a majority of people, although adapting each individual diet to account for differences in metabolism and body type, this is a concise approach that can act as a point of departure.

Once you wake up in the morning, your organism is basically "strong" since most people sleep for about 6 to 8 hours a day. In 6 to 8 hours, when the body is denied food, the body begins to use stored energy sources. To maintain constant blood sugar and to power the brain and other tissues during sleep.

The body slowly sends out nutrients from the liver, fat cells, and muscle cells. The body may use glycogen stored for energy (if you have eaten it properly to optimize glycogen storage, only minimal destruction of the body's cells (due to the incapacity of the body to store amino acids). The best thing you can do for your body is to use a relatively rapidly digested protein source when you wake.

A whey protein or protein hydrolysate shake is your best bet since it takes just 20 minutes to lift the blood amino acid level before almost all you eat flows through your bloodstream, and somewhere between 20 and 40 minutes to hit its high point. This is accompanied by a standard breakfast meal consisting of a low-fat protein source of high quality and low glycemic carbohydrates.

Protein consumption During day

Because you want to eat small, simple meals every few hours throughout the day, the need for "extra" proteins is minimal. My preference is high-quality low-fat protein products and low-glycemic carbohydrates or a good protein blend. When you can't eat a good meal every two hours with a good mixture of whey / casein / milk protein and focus, the combination of strong proteins and a slow protein can be a good compromise.

Protein Intake Shortly before training

If you have a small number of foods throughout the day, "extra" proteins from non-food sources would not be required. But if you miss a meal and decide to practice in 60 minutes than a fast protein, like whey protein hydrolysate, glutamines, and branched-chain amino acids, you need easy digestion.

A fluid meal containing protein and carbohydrates that increase the amount of insulin (an anabolic hormone, increasing the absorption of amino acid and glucose into your muscle) one hour before training. Amino acids of the ramified chain promote protein synthesis.

You can use the complete proteins to heal by adding additional Baca items that are ingested during the workout. The body will absorb extra branch-chain amino acids from the full proteins, which will make the rest of the protein incomplete and unusable for developing.

The user of a liquid meal that includes protein and carbohydrates one hour before exercise can increase insulin (an anabolic hormone that increases the intake in the muscles of amino acids and glucose).

Protein consumption Shortly after exercise

The most important meal of the day is the meal shortly after your training (don't listen to other people telling you that your breakfast is). The post-working meal is very important because the body is especially sensitive to the consumption of nutrients. Normally, blood amino and blood insulin levels are lower.

Due to the lower levels of blood amino acids, it is an important time for rapid digestion of fast protein, such as whey protein hydrolysates, to keep your body in healthy nitrogen balance and anabolic condition. Hydrolyzed proteins have a higher biological value than concentrates or other protein preparations, usually suggesting a greater protein use in the body. Higher proteins of biological value may also increase the release of IGF-1 that can promote muscle growth. The cell's intense hunger and the fast action properties of the whey ensure that you use the best window to recover fully. Instead, the body chases the accumulated nutrient stores, and, in the case of a diet, it, for example, robs other muscle tissues of glutamine.

A minimum amount of high-glycemic carbohydrates (e.g., maltodextrin and dextrose), quickly digested, should also be eaten with the post-workout whey protein meal to optimize the full intake of protein and glycogen content.

Note: With this post-training meal, adding high glycemic index carbohydrates induces strong and rapid increases in glycogen insulin and also stimulates the synthesis. Creatine and glutamine can also help you heal afterward. Fat slows digestion, and the supply of nutrients should also provide minimum fat content. You will eat this meal within 60 minutes of your weight training.

Protein intake after exercise, but before the last meal My preferences are to eat low-quality fat protein foods (such as chicken breast, turkey breast, etc.) and low-glycemic carbohydrates (such as fibrous vegetables, brown rice...). Consumption of a food-protein meal can also inhibit muscle breakdown levels by reducing amino acid releases through the body. Carbohydrates should also be included in this meal to stimulate insulin release. Insulin is also a hormone that controls the rate of protein synthesis. Increasing insulin release can slow the rate of muscle breakdown.

Protein consumption Most often found to be fabulous right before bedtime.
People believe that fat preservation is encouraged. My personal belief is that if you want to maintain muscle mass, it is important that you eat right before retirement, to prevent the body from using all its stored energy at night. Because at least six hours you will not have another meal, this meal will contain a slow protein, which releases nutrients over several hours.

Carb timing

In this order, the two most important foods are post-training and breakfast. These are ideal times for carbohydrates (for a 200-pound bodybuilder, 90–100 g carbohydrates at breakfast are used to restore liver and muscle glycogen and to promote protein synthesis, preventing catabolism (muscle waste) and minimizing the risk of your carbohydrates turning into body fat).

Start your day with Carbs (Conditional).

Besides the post-meal, breakfast is another golden time to eat carbs since your blood sugar and muscle glycogen levels are low at night quickly. The body has to fill these amounts before fat storage machinery is activated in the body.

Consume Organic High Glycemic Index Foods high in the Glycemic index at the right time,

but their intake should not be completely blocked. High glycemic natural foods can be helpful. For starters, fruits contain beneficial nutrients and fiber, so balance is important. When eating small amounts of fruit, you can sometimes obtain the beneficial nutrients and fibers while reducing the possible adverse effects of high fructose intake.

Recall that controlling the consumption of carbohydrates provides many benefits such as reducing the risk of heart attack, reducing stored body fat, and reducing the risk of insulin resistance from cells. The effective control of the consumption of carbohydrates involves understanding food timing as well as what food will adversely affect the endocrine system if consumed excessively — learning how the Glycemic Index functions are also important for controlling blood insulin levels effectively.

After exercise, Eat simple carbs IMMEDIATELY

Fast-acting carbs (those with a high Glycemic index) can increase insulin levels, reduce muscle catabolism, and promote increased metabolism. This post-training meal should be eaten in 30 minutes and not later than 1 hour after the end of the training.

The meal should consist of approximately 75 grams of bodyweight carbs (150 grams for 200 pounds of men), with a 50% (75 grams) of carbohydrates derived from high-glycemic, easy-to-down sources such as white rice, wheat crème, mash potatoes, etc. High glycaemic carbs are easily digested from non-fibrous soft textured carbs, which result in a rapid insulin reaction that leads to the production of amino acids-the building blocks of muscle tissue-and encourages anabolism. Note: Consider reducing this amount to about half to 75% during the pre-contest time.

Eat the Carbs Majority Upon exercise,

Eat a smaller carbohydrate meal to facilitate the preparation. It must be low enough that the cardiovascular session is carbohydrates to burn fat. Your biggest carbohydrate meal should be on your post-training meal, as it will be saved as fat less likely, as your body will use it to refill your exercise and cardio lessons with depleting glycogen. This meal will take about 25 percent of your daily carbs. This should amount to approximately 150 grams of carbs for a 200-pound individual (during the pre-campaign period, the proportion of the total calories and the total grams of carbs ingested are reduced).

Avoid Carbs After Hours

If a super-fast metabolism does not harm you, you should forget to eat baked potatoes late in the night. Late-night carbohydrates interfere with growth hormone release and promote fat storage while you sleep.

Don't Let your Energy Control You

As a kid, energy is continually flowing. In fact, some children are "treated" for their energy abundance. Yet as we age, our energy levels seem to decline, and we just want to have the energy we've had as adolescents. Sadly, stress, exhaustion, poor nutrition, sleep deprivation, overtime work, mental barriers, and many other factors all lead to decreased levels of energy. What we don't know is that we control our own levels of energy. Energy shortage is a self-inflicted disease (if you like). We need to get back to the fundamentals of life as we used to be children and revive our constantly fluid youth fountain.

Think about it when you were a child, you didn't have a care in the world, you enjoyed life, and you absorbed all the information. You have experienced life at a time. You've probably eaten more healthy food than before, you have gone to bed early, you've eaten breakfast, you've smiled, you've laughed, you have hopes and dreams, you're involved, you are airy, you've only had sugar on a birthday party. Recall all that you loved had a passion for and learned as a child... Are not most of them stuff you should bring into your lives today?

I'm going to help you on the right path. Next, delete from your diet all unwanted sugars. Sugar is body medicine. The bodies were not designed to take processed and refined sugar, and carbohydrate-preserved food. Remember what your mother told you always? Eat green beans! Actually, eat as much natural, unprocessed, healthy food as you can. The body is intended to feed foods that are grown in the land or from a tree, foods derived from animals and animal fats. This functions more effectively if the body is supplied with foods that can break down. Be watchful for food labels as sucre may appear in anything (ketchup, dressing in salads, crackers). Eliminating sugar will activate your body, which will increase energy levels, replenish undernourished cells, and naturally balance your systems. Fat loss could actually be an added benefit.

With more energy from your dietary improvements, you can feel more involved. Activity is a natural stimulant for the body... in certain parameters. Power workout. Just 20-30 minutes per day with strength training and cardiovascular exercise as part of your program. Training for more than 45 minutes a day will lead to energy loss, as the body will start drawing energy from your protein reserves (that is muscle!) Training causes the body to release endorphins (which are "feel-good" hormones) that leave you with a normal after-effect. Concentrate on improving body strength by exercises of body weight. Completing many push-ups, pull-ups, squats, and seating-ups can be a struggle to get going. There is no need for gym membership. Concentrate on improving the natural function of the body before taking more demanding practice plans. As with any workout scheme, take one day a week off from your exercise completely to allow the body to return to 100 percent strength.

Food quality is not only a key factor in energy production but also nutrition timing. Can you remember your mother's supper ready to eat after a long day out, or at least a wholesome snack? What she did not realize is that she contributed from a full day of exercise to your low energy levels by re-alimenting your body instantly. Try to eat the greatest meal or workout after the day. Eating within an hour is essential for the recovery of your body and the energy level of the next day. Muscles are broken down during an intense workout or aerobic training (that is, muscle soreness), and food is needed as a fuel source for those cells to begin to regenerate in order to help these muscles recover more quickly and stronger. This helps not only speed up the recovery process but also avoids soreness in the following days.

Sleep is another major factor I listed in the introductory paragraph. When it runs 7-8 hours of sleep (for most people), the body is best revitalized. It is recommended that you get to bed by 10 p.m. because the body sleeps most well during the time between 11 p.m. and 2 a.m. Therefore hit the sack by ten or 22:30 to make the best use of your sleep schedule. Another reason to sleep well is that both the brain and the body fill up. When a person is tired, the body craves energy for carbohydrates (i.e., sugar!), despite being the last source of energy that it requires, which causes insulin rushes and crashes, making the problem even worse. So get to bed at 10 pm, and all else runs smoothly.

One final item for increased energy is intermittent fasting. For adults, we tend to think we have to eat at 8 a.m. because that's what breakfast is served, and if we are hungry or not, we have to eat at noon because lunch is always served, and we have to eat again at 5 p.m. for the same usual reason. This is all well and good, but most of us have a break where we have coffee and a snack, hungry or not. Some go so far as to have an afternoon snack in front of the bed, which is a big no, as it interferes with our restful sleep from 10 am to 2 pm. The body will try to break down the excess of sugar we eat before closing our eyes for the night, which does not fully allow our system to rest. But sometimes, when we overeat or drink a high glycemic burden of a food, our bodies need to digest the food longer. Furthermore, high sugar meals can lead to other symptoms, such as bloating, vomiting, nausea, headaches, joint inflammation, etc., which take more than four to five hours before returning to normal. Fasting 12-18 hours a day (or whenever you eat over food) is therefore a good way for the body to return naturally to its normal working state. It produces more strength by loading the body with food, blocking its natural flow, and cleaning up or detoxifying the liver and bloodstream of nutrients.

So if you want more energy, consider these recommendations as part of your daily scheme. Take one or two pieces of advice and get them to work for you. I believe you'll see a difference in how you feel and how your body works. We must all return to the basics of life and remember what our youthful conduct was behind! It could be your motivation to help yourself.

Chapter Five:
How to Setup an Intermittent Fasting Diet

Welcome to Fasting 101 periodic. This is a first, or reference to the system I myself use for weight loss intermittent fasting.

This is a clear description of how it works:

- Eat 9 hours a day during training days, and fast 15 hours the rest.
- Take 6 hours a day off, or cardio days, and quickly take the remaining 18.
- Cardio 2-4 times a week
- Maintenance + 500 calories on weight training days
- Maintaining 50% of the maintenance on other days
- Most carbohydrate consumption is in weight training days Again, this plan is unique to fat loss.
- Weight training three days a week
- Plans must soon be made for mass gain (bulking) and repair.

Fasting Times/Establishing Eating

Now for the detailed explanation: how to set up an irregular fat-loss diet that determines eating times. The time of day you eat depends on whether or not you lift weights that day. The feeding cycle lasts 9 hours on days off or exercise, and 6 hours on days off or cardio. You will have to be in a position to weight the train and cardio on the schedule at the same time of day.

Eating schedule for weight training days

The fast is interrupted by a pre-workout shake 15-30 minutes before you are working and lasts for 9 hours. Nutrition routine for weight training days Because I work out at 1:00, for example, my eating period starts at 12:30 and continues until 9:30 pm. If you do training at 8 pm, then I find the weightlifting is better at lunch or in the morning.

First, we should consider setting up a holiday or cardio plan.

Eating schedule for off or cardio days

One hour after cardio is done and lasts 6 hours, and fast is interrupted. I cardio at 1 pm in my case, so my pace is interrupted at 15 pm. It remains in the afternoon at 3 pm.

Description

Since I'm practicing Monday / Wednesday / Friday, the picture seems like this:

Monday: Fast ends at 12:30 pm and starts at 9:30 pm

Tuesday, Fast finishes at 3 pm and begins at 21:00 pm

Wednesday, Fast terminates at 12:30 pm and begins at 21:30 the

Thursday, Fast ends at 3:00 pm

Friday, and starts at 21:00 pm, I know that at first, with all the mathematics, this might seem daunting, but once you first define your criteria, it's quite simple and routine.

Calories available for Fat Loss Calorie requirements depend on whether it's a day of weight training or an off / cardio day only.

To calculate calories needed for fat loss, the calories necessary for maintenance must first be determined. The easiest way to measure your weight is to raise by 15 pounds. For starters, if you weigh 200 lbs, you need 3000 calories a day to sustain them.

Calorie requirements for weight training days:

Take the amount of maintenance calories and add 500 to calorie determination on weight training days. So for our 200 lb guy, on days they raise, they will eat 3500 calories.

Calorie requirement on off or cardio days:

Simply divide your maintenance calories into half in order to determine calories needed for off or cardio days. Our 200 lb person would, therefore, eat 1500 calories per day for off or aerobic days.

Macronutrient Breakdown:

Now that you have calculated your calorie needs for fat loss, it is time to figure out how many macronutrients you will need.

Macronutrient breakdown:

Fat: the average amount of fat consumed every day is 30 grams; the amount varies whether you weigh that day or not.

The macronutrients that we will use will be the great three:

* Fat

* Protein

* Carbohydrates

(Remember that fat has nine calories per gram and protein and carbs each have four calories per g.). Where the fat comes from, doesn't matter, as long as ten of these grams are in the form of omega-3 fish oil.

Protein: You multiply your weight by 1.25 to determine the minimum amount of protein per day. Our 200 lb person needs at least 250 g of protein for muscle preservation. Definitions don't matter, just make sure you don't hit the fat cap. Eggs, very lean red meat, free fat cheese, and protein powder (whey or casein) are great choices.

Carbohydrates: The remaining calories in your diet are carbohydrates. Once, don't matter, just make sure you don't exceed the 30 g fat cap and keep your sugar below 100 g. So he receives 270 calories from fat in our sample individual and 1000 calories from protein. With the caloric target of 3500 days, he has 2230 calories remaining for carbohydrates. Divide 2230 by four and yield a maximum of~558 grams of carbohydrate.

Non-lifting or cardio-days macronutrient breakdown: As I said earlier, calories needed during days when you don't train to weight or cardio are 1/2 of what your maintenance calories are. Here's the macronutrient breakdown: Fat: Again, from training days, the amount of fat is unchanged. The maximum fat consumed per day is 30 grams. Where the fat comes from, it doesn't matter, as long as 10 of those grams are in the Omega-3 Fish Oil form.

Carbohydrates: Carbohydrate sources should only come from fibrous green vegetables on rest days or cardio-only for days, and trace amounts found in the sources of your protein such as whey and cheese. The maximum daily amount should not exceed 20 grams.

Protein: the minimum protein amount is your pounds weight of 1.25. For our sample person who has 1500 calories a day, he will obtain 270 fat calories, 80 carbohydrate calories, and 1,150 protein calories. The equivalent would be ~287.5 grams.

Weight Training Days diet Weight Training Days are a full-body regimen three days a week. I use Monday-Wednesday-Friday myself, but the days are up for you as long as there is a day off between activities. Continue to read my exercise review.

Pre-workout The strong is disrupted by a whey protein/carb shake on training days 15-30 minutes before the workout starts.

I propose a mixture of simple carbs and whey protein.

Protein=.25 g / lbx weight Carbs=.25 g / lbx weight My pre-workout carb is my preference. I have no pre-made liquid form. Keep fat here to a minimum.

You have another shake in 30 minutes of your training but use the whey + casein/dextrose mix.

Protein=.25g / lbx weight Carbs=.50g / lbx weight Rest of the day The first good daily meal will be 1 hour after PWO. This will be the day's greatest meal. You have to feed the rest of the time. However, I suggest adding your calories to your last meal. Remember that you don't have to eat every 2-3 hours with Intermittent Fasting. Only ensure that your caloric/macronutrient goals are achieved. I still prescribe a casein shake just before the eating time has finished. Since it's a slow protein to digest, it will allow you to hold it longer.

Off or cardio days diet Because calories are significantly reduced during off or cardio days, the eating period is shorter. This works best for 2-3 good meals instead of 6-7, as you read in muscle mags.

For cardio days, a 50 g protein shake breaks up easily, 1 hour after cardio is complete. After two hours, have your first "actual" meal and keep going for 6 hours. As I said earlier, carbs are limited to 20 a day and will consist of fibrous green vegetables and food traces.

Weight Training Regimen Weight Training is a full-body 3-day regimen. Also, exact dates are not really important, just make sure you have a day off between workouts. On days 1 and 2, you just work large muscles (legs, back, chest) and incorporate arms/calves into the smaller muscle on day 3. For each large muscle, you make four sets of 6-8 reps and 2-3 sets of 8-12 reps for the smaller ones.

Day 1: Push Flat Bench Pressen / Shoulder Press / Leg Press / Weighted Crunches
Day 2: Pull Rows / Chinups / Hamstring Curl
Day 3: Push / Pull Incline Bench Press / Rows / Squats / Calf Rises / Barbell Curl / Lateral Raise /Lateral lift / Tricep Pushdown / Back Extensions / Weighted Crunches.
The exercise must be down 2-3 days a week to maximum fat loss. Start warming up for 5 minutes and then start training at a high-intensity period of 10 minutes. It works best on an elliptical or a spinning cycle rather than a treadmill. You will do this in an interval of 1 minute. One minute high strength followed by a 1-minute moderate pace. Repeat until it's

up to 10 minutes. Drink some water and relax for five minutes after the HIIT session is over. Upon your rest, do the steady State Cardio 30 minutes of low to moderate strength. A treadmill works fantastically for this. Don't forget to have your 50 g of protein and wait an hour.

Nutritional Tips to Burn Fat

I shall give you five convenient tips to make your body a fat-burning tool- you should take information with you and practice every day, both inside and outside the fitness center or workout area. Instead of quantifying specific amounts, I will give you a few simple ideas.

Eat Fiber

Come to the right thing. A high fiber diet will minimize fat and cholesterol absorption in your intestines (preventing accumulation of fat), delay the absorption of glucose in the bloodstream (which means more sugar is consumed with energy, less is stored with fat), regulate insulin levels and hinder the emptying of your stomach (which will both decrease your appetite), and make your body entirely stronger (so you eat less). Evidence has shown that low fat, high fiber diet results in almost three times the weight loss of a low fiber diet. So how are you getting your fiber? Here is how I get mine:
One salad fully loaded, one oat cup, and 2-3 raw fruits a day (fruit bonus: Citrus vitamin can also be beneficial in burning fat).

Eat Calcium

Research shows that three to four daily portions of low-fat milk products will lead to body fat reduction. Higher calcium levels stored in fat cells may contribute to a decrease in fat and induce an increase in thermogenesis (the core temperature of the body). The most appropriate calcium is obtained from dairy products such as low-fat milk, yogurt, and cottage cheese. Other good sources include salmon, dark leafy vegetables, oats, and almonds, particularly for the lactose intolerant (note the additional fiber bonus).

Eat Breakfast

Breakfast is the most important meal of the day. Studies have shown that people with big, nutritious breakfasts lose considerably more fat than people they miss coffee. They avoid breakfast. Coffee is not going to help you spill extra pounds. Instead, it can lead to loss of muscle and decreases in metabolism, which prevents your ability to burn fat. A big glass of water, fresh fruit, a bowl of oatmeal, and nuts, is a great example of breakfast. Also remember: if it isn't nutritious, breakfast will work against you, too. Fried meats, sweet muffins, and croissants, sugar-filled cereals, or packaged packaging do not count as a healthy breakfast!

Eat Frequently

Feed Frequently A million times ago, you've read it: 5-6 meals a day are better than three meals. I would like to take that a step further, depending on your energy consumption and needs, up to 10 times a day or more. Examples (from my personal food log) are: 1) banana 7 am; 2) oatmeal 9 am; 3) handful of almonds 10:30am; 4) three slices of turkey 12 pm; 5) yogurt 1 pm; 6) apple 14 pm; 7) big salad 4:30 pm; 8) protein bar 7:00 pm; 9) handful grapes 8:15pm; 10) 1 spinach scramble egg 9 pm (both at 11 pm). The theory behind eating is that the physical effect of digestion has a metabolism, so you maintain a higher metabolism rate by constantly feeding them. So long, so the pasture is safe, more calories are consumed throughout the day. On the other hand, eating too seldom causes the body to go hungry and conserve energy, resulting in increased fat accumulation, and a lower digestive and overall metabolism.

Eat Water

The studies have shown that the muscles are less involved, and the metabolism is dropping and that the body consumes fat more efficiently without sufficient water. A slight reduction in metabolism will add up to more than 10 pounds of fat a year! Water also tends to curb your appetite and give you a "full feeling." So, you can drink a few glasses of water every day, drink a glass of water 30 minutes before your workout, drink water daily in the fitness center, and drink water after the workout (speed up your recovery too!). Most natural foods such as fruit and vegetables (and protein, vitamins, minerals, phytonutrients, etc.) are also high in water content. This is another wonderful way to get your H2O.

This chapter will give you five more tips that will make your body a fat-burning machine that builds up lean muscle. If you did not read the last five recommendations, the summary consisted of increasing the fiber intake, always drinking water, consuming a complex and balanced breakfast, increasing the amount of calcium, and having a few small meals per day (up to 8-10). Ready for more? Ready for more? Good! Good! Continue reading...

#6: Eat carbs early in the day Meals containing larger carbohydrate levels should be consumed earlier in the day. It means you can eat all of your whole grain and fruit before noon. The metabolism of your body is highest earlier in the day, so this is a great time for your muscles to supply Glycogen nutrition (carbohydrates), thus retaining many of the nutrients carbs you consume are fuel consumed instead of stored as fat stores. Most families tend to have the biggest dinner of the day, typically when the body needs the least energy and the metabolism is lowest. For reality, breakfast would be bigger, and dinner would be smaller. And seek-prioritize consuming carbohydrates early in the day and concentrate on raising the portion size of carbohydrates as the afternoon and evening progress.

#7: Eat the correct kind of carbohydrates Though carbohydrates are essential to supply energy, and allow your body to burn fat, choose the right carbohydrates. Easy carbohydrates like sugar and processed food, such as fat deposition-insulin, are quickly absorbed into the digestive system. In addition, the quick release of energy followed by a fast drop in the levels of sugar can cause you to want more food, so many people on a standard US diet are* still* hungry! No matter which percentage of your diet consists of carbohydrates, you must choose slowly absorbing and digested complex carbohydrates and create a long-term source of energy that keeps you more satisfied for a longer period.

Wholesale grain flours, beans, oats, and unprocessed seeds, including brown or wild rice, are a great choice and include many other compounds essential for maintaining the proper digestive function and high metabolism.

#8 Eat fat Mainstream Americans have shifted over the last few decades to low fat or no diet, usually resulting in* increased* obesity and chronic disease and decreased health and fitness. Meanwhile, animal populations such as Eskimos, which eat up to 70% of their diet in whale and fish fat calories, have one of the lowest rates of cardiac disease in the world. There are some very good reasons, though this may seem ironic. Carbohydrate consumption usually increases to replace calories not supplied by dietary fat. The increased consumption of carbohydrates contributes to a higher fat burn, which appears to contribute to blood sugar absorption, the use of muscle tissue as food, low energy, and lower metabolism and the production of hormones. Therefore, many Americans would replace saturated fat, like butter, with trans fat, like margarine. For the body, trans fats are far worse than saturated fat. It is, therefore, necessary to select the right type of fat. Cholesterol is present in the majority of animal fats and vegetable oils, which leads to cardiac disease. Nonetheless, monounsaturated fats, such as olive oil, nuts, fish oil, and various seed oils, may lead to lower cholesterol, lower the risk of heart disease and increase the body's capacity for fuel-burning fat. So, try eating fish a few days a week (or adding fish oil), cook with olive oil, and try eating at least a handful of a good nut (e.g., almonds or walnuts) once a day.

#9 Avoid replacements for Chemical sugar sweeteners, like aspartame, always taste sweet (so it's sugar substitution!). Once your tongue's taste receptors detect this sweet material, your digestive system creates compounds that prepare your body to absorb the "food" your brain thinks you are consuming. The hormones produced by your digestive process are still present once this fake nourishment gets into your small intestine, but it does not actually release energy or satiety, which leaves you with an intestine full of digestive hormones and needs food to break down. This is why studies have shown that diet soda intake is linked to obesity! If you are serious about burnished fat, say any foods or dietary drinks substituting sugar that you currently eat. I guarantee you can feel a hundred times better once you've experienced the initial relapse of addiction.

CARBS, FAT, AND PROTEIN FOR ATHLETES

For preparation and recovery, some coaches and nutritionists recommend complex carbohydrates, whereas others recommend both simple and complex carbohydrates. Although simple sugar like chocolate, high-fructose corn syrup, or glucose is indeed processed into the body more easily, this isn't necessarily a good thing. The body's response to simple sugars involves a rapid rise in blood sugar levels, followed by a decrease in sugar levels or a hypoglycemic response. An endurance athlete who uses single carbohydrates during training or race can, therefore, undergo multiple spikes and subsequent decreases in blood sugar levels. This should not be an issue for an endurance event of 60 minutes or less. Nevertheless, since the event extends this time period, such as an ironman sprint, more complex carbohydrates at a pace of about 30-60 grams per hour should be consumed. For such cases, Hammer Gel, a supplier of endurance athletes, offers a big, complex carbohydrate gel, as do other manufacturers. Obviously, simple sugars eaten at any time other than a breed can potentially lead to increased deposition of fatty body, decreased metabolism, and generally poor health, so restrict your intake to quick, intense rides—note, try it during your training before trying in a breed!

As far as proteins are concerned, I would like to zero in the protein source of branched-chain amino acids (BCAA). The body relies on protein as a source of fuel for training that is extremely intense or lasts longer than three hours. Leucine, isoleucine, and valine are BCAAs and can satisfy the energy requirements by up to 10 percent. These can be bought at many health food stores or gyms as supplements and are also used in several commercial endurance gels. Most dairy products, whey protein, and red meat are a natural source. Isoleucine is present in most foodstuffs and is abundant in meats, fish, and cheese; in foodstuffs like beans, brewer's yeast, rice bran, caseinate, and corn; and valin food sources include soy meal, cottage cheese, pork, wheat, champagne and peanuts, meats and plants.

BCAAs should be used during heavy lifting, strength endurance cycles (closer to race season), and high altitude training. Of note, only three of the many amino acids the body needs for regeneration and tissue growth are BCAAs, therefore do not rely on them as the sole source of protein.

Fat is, of course, a very powerful long-term source of energy. For longer races, one form of fat, medium-chain triglycerides, has proven to increase stamina and speed. The body absorbs medium-chain triglycerides quicker for use as energy and less likely to be retained as body fat. Once again, medium-chain triglycerides from various manufacturers of sports supplements and health food stores are available. Coconut oil is a growing and increasingly popular natural source. Remember that the consumption of these fats on an empty stomach can lead to a rather irritating gastrointestinal distress.

Nutritional Strategies for Fitness Success

Nutrition and rest are frequently the disregarded components of work out schedules, and the principle reason that such a significant number of neglect to understand their objectives. Such a large number of individuals attempt to out-exercise a poor diet and poor rest propensities, which is an unimaginable activity while expecting to get results. At irrefutably the most, individuals may wind up training for 5 hours every week (for the vast majority 3-4 hours per seven days stretch of appropriate training is bounty).

There are 168 hours inconsistently. It is difficult to imagine that you can train hard for 3-5 hours out of each week, and afterward disregard what you do the staying 163 hours of the week, and expect to get results.

What number of CALORIES SHOULD I EAT?

If you are attempting to lose fat, set your day by day calories at 12 times your body weight

If you are attempting to pick up muscle, eat 16 times your body weight in calories day by day

Try not to get excessively got up to speed in tallying calories; however, because what you eat and when you eat, it could compare to carefully checking what number of calories you eat.

The amount of PROTEIN SHOULD I EAT?

Attempt to eat 1 gram of protein for each pound of body weight every day. Protein intake is important for various reasons:

It is the structure squares of muscle; without it, your body will be not able to fix the harm you do through your training. It is additionally muscle saving when on a calorie decreased eating regimen for fat loss.

What that fundamentally means is that sufficient protein intake will keep your body from separating muscle tissue for vitality necessities when you are lessening your calorie intake to burn fat.

More muscle rises to more calories burned at rest since the body burns a larger number of calories significantly to keep up muscle than it does look after fat. By chance, this is one reason it is difficult to lose excess body fat, as it is a useful put-away crisis fuel for times that the body doesn't get enough calories for its day by day vitality needs.

The human body is programmed to sacrifice muscle and extra fat for survival. This is why diet and nutrition is such an essential part of any wellness or fat loss program.

WHEN SHOULD I EAT CARBOHYDRATES?

On training days, keep your carbohydrate intake low during the day except in the wake of training.

On non-training days, attempt to keep your carbohydrate intake to under 30 yet not over 50 grams (or as near this as would be prudent).

Carbohydrates spike your insulin levels, and insulin is a capacity hormone. If you are spiking your insulin levels throughout the day, whatever isn't burned off will be put away either as muscle or as fat for later vitality.

If you spike your insulin levels after an exercise and give a lot of protein, this will be put away in your muscles and won't bring on any significant fat addition.

If you spike insulin some other time, any excess will be put away as body fat.

Examples of carbohydrate consumption, as per exercise plan:

TRAINING DAYS:

- Carbs around 150 grams, devoured simply in the wake of training (however much as could reasonably be expected)
- Approximately 1 gram of protein for each pound of bodyweight
- Calories = Bodyweight x 12 - 16

NON-TRAINING DAYS:

- Carbs under 30 grams
- Meals to comprise of protein and fats
- Approximately 1 gram of protein for every pound of bodyweight
- Calories = Bodyweight x 12 - 16

A viable, and reasonable, technique for controlling your carbohydrate consumption for fat loss is called carb cycling, which is nitty-gritty beneath:

- DAY 1 and 2 - No Carbs
- DAY 3 - Refeed
- DAY 4 and 5 - No Carbs
- DAY 6 and 7 - Refeed

The refeed days are significant for various reasons.

To begin with, it is simpler mentally to adhere to a program this way if you realize you get the opportunity to cheat the following two days.

Besides, if you abandon carbs for over six days at the total max, hormones, for example, leptin, which is a central point in fat burning, will get messed up, and your body will store body fat because it is in survival mode.

REST and RECOVERY

Rest and recuperation are real parts of any work out schedule. Training is just the boost that you give your body to change, yet if you are not eating appropriately and getting enough rest, your body won't most likely fix and improve itself.

Rest is essential as this is the place muscles are made, and fat is burned. If you train hard (and intelligent) and eat right, your body will develop and fix itself while you rest. The ideal measure of rest is 7-8 hours consistently, yet attempt to get as much as your lifestyle and wellbeing permits.

Rest is additionally the time when growth hormone emission is the most astounding. Growth hormone is fundamentally in charge of muscle growth and fix, yet it likewise affects fat burning.

Insufficient rest equivalents lower levels of growth hormone and a debilitating level of fat burning. Lack of sleep has likewise been connected in numerous studies to higher rates of obesity.

WHAT IS INTERMITTENT FASTING?

Intermittent Fasting is a nutritional system that looks to maximize the body's capacity to burn fat. Rather than having breakfast (which isn't the most important feast of the day, in opposition to prevalent thinking), you would eat your first supper of the day around noon or presently.

You would then eat mostly protein/fats during the rest of the day (subject to your caloric necessities), with by far most of your carbohydrate intake and calories eaten after your training.

Numerous studies demonstrate that growth hormones and different hormones ideal for fat loss are higher in a fasted state. If you are going fast for the initial segment of your day, you are empowering your body to burn body fat as fuel, which will prompt higher rates of fat loss, generally speaking.

If, nonetheless, you attempt intermittent Fasting and find that it is expanding your desires for awful nourishments, for example, doughnuts, and so on, it is likely better over the long haul to have a morning meal comprising of for the most part protein and fats, yet not carbohydrates.

You can, in any case, get a large portion of the advantages of Fasting if you can delay your morning meal in any event 2 hours after you wake up.

Remember that there is a time of modification that will happen over time of half a month while your body changes and becomes accustomed to burning fat as fuel.

WHAT KINDS OF FOOD SHOULD I EAT?

Continuously attempt to get the sustenances you eat as natural and normally nourished as conceivable as this will limit hormones, chemicals, pesticides, herbicides, and so forth.

Protein:
- Whole natural eggs
- Organic grass nourished hamburger
- Chicken
- Pork
- Bacon
- Cheese

- Cottage cheese
- Sour cream
- Wild got fish
- Tuna
- Whole or crude milk

Fats:

- Virgin, cold squeezed coconut oil
- Virgin olive oil (be exceptionally mindful to avoid vegetable oils, for example, canola and soybean oil as they are prepared to utilize chemical and high heat and advance irritation in the body.
- Unprocessed regular spread (without included shading)
- Nuts/seeds (make sure to part out appropriately, as nuts can push you over your calorie targets effectively as they are very calorie thick)

Carbohydrates:

- Rice
- Potatoes
- Yams
- Quinoa
- Pasta
- Bananas or different organic products
- Tortilla wraps
- Bread

When having a grain affectability (the same number of individuals do nowadays), clearly stay away from it, yet bread is not a terrible decision of carbohydrate post-exercise as I would like to think and experience.

Most thing isn't 100% awful for you and could be valuable if utilized at the correct times and sums. The equivalent can be said for pasta or other defamed carbohydrates; timing and cycling them is the way to using them successfully.

Different CONSIDERATIONS

Figure out how to peruse nutrition names, and considerably more importantly, fixing names. Such a significant number of sustenances considered "solid" have an extensive rundown of unfortunate chemicals and fixings in them.

A decent general guideline is to keep away from handled nourishment (anything that arrives in a box can or pack), however much as could reasonably be expected. Additionally, avoid margarine and anything that has a TV ad or similar ad. Avoid artificial sugars and pop.

It is a smart thought to eat your last feast of the day comprising for the most of protein, before bed (mainly if you are intermittent Fasting), as your body will utilize them to reimbursed your muscle tissue while you are resting. Some significant decisions incorporate entire eggs, cottage cheese, plain Greek yogurt, and so on.

You are permitted to eat as many greens and crisp, crude vegetables as you like. Attempt to join them into each feast. Attempt to limit natural product consumption to after your training, as the sugar levels will spike your insulin levels, which stops fat burning.

Only cleanliness things, for example, antiperspirant, aroma, cologne, and so forth, are likewise things to watch out for. They frequently contain chemicals that can upset thyroid yield and hormone levels/creation in the body, prompting higher estrogen levels and fat addition. Chemicals utilized in canned merchandise can contain chemicals, for example, this too.

Intermittent Fasting And The Phase 1 Diet For Maximum Fat Burning

Most readers may only be Well connected to one or the other. Both of them have a unique style, which packs a big punch too fat loss and health. On the surface, only one is regarded as a "diet," but even this term is very loose. I am familiar with both in terms of fat loss and overall health benefits so that an objective overview is appropriate for both of them. I really think that if you bridge the gap and combine these two forms, you will bring about some impressive fat loss performance. Let's start! Let's start!

The concept of fasting in a diet plan appears to get very negative comments within the fitness community. Fasting for fat loss is extremely effective. Most companies and coaches claim that if you do not eat every few hours, the metabolism will slow or make our bodies go to "Hunger." Before we go any further, we must remember that "slowing down the metabolism" may be one of the biggest misconceptions in the fitness industry. The metabolism of chronic low-calorie consumption declines over the last weeks. This is not when you fly a few days a week. Here is a clear description of how sporadic quicking is applied to someone's schedule. I'm going to explain how this can be changed later.

1. Usually eat until dinner (2-4 meals, not 6-8)
2. Eat your dinner, but then stop eating.
3. Quick before the next day's dinner. (No calorie intake)
4. Eat a daily dinner for that night.

You still fly for a 24-hour cycle in this method but still have a meal every day. This is usually done 1-2 days a week. You will easily drop a lot of weight three days a week before a holiday or a meeting. For only a few weeks, I'd suggest this.

What you know about yourself through fasting

You want to mention some changes in the way you eat. Once you have finished your 24-hour fast a few times, when, when, and why you eat can be revealed to you. Many of the reasons why we eat are due to emotional ties or mere behaviors and not real hunger itself. Sometimes we are so ready to eat that when we are not hungry, we consume a meal.

Fasting on time is a lifestyle, not a diet

It does not limit you to certain foods, recettes, ratios, rules, or charts to follow in order to lose weight. This makes your obsessive-compulsive eating habits and helps you to enjoy the variety. Instead of avoiding a certain food completely because someone has told you, you simply will not over-eat any kind of "evil" food by adding a number of foods. Now that this field of fat loss has been established, let us turn to a deeper problem in food and health.

What is the first diet process AKA The Fungus Link?

Doug Kaufmann is the founder of the theory that fungi and yeast lead to poor health and weight loss. He has studied and reported how fungi produce toxic substances known as "mycotoxins" that cause many health problems. This addresses the problem by treating areas where fungi and yeast can enter the body, but also offers a way to kill the disease in order to reverse the effects of so many medical conditions in America. He found that fungi want different carbohydrates, like humans. The understanding that fungi require carbohydrates to survive inside the body makes it understandable to use phase 1 diet.

So, what is the Phase 1 Diet Allowed?

This is the only "diet" I recommend that simply limits all food types, but for a particular reason. Many foods are temporarily omitted in order to starve and destroy bacteria and to expose the origin of food cravings. Uncontrolled food cravings can harm your health and the addition of pounds in the abdomen, thighs, hips, you name. Overgrowth of the fungus may potentially be the root failure to lose weight. You will continue to eat and eat unattended as long as you are addicted to certain foods. Most people see their wellbeing as strong as it can't believe how amazing they look. A great reason for this is the specific food choice that hungers and avoids fungal overcrowding. Most people are better at feeding because of this breakdown. Here is a quick overview of food choices appropriate to the Phase 1 diet.

Example:

Acceptable foods for step

1,) eggs

2) FROUCH: beers, grapefruit, limon, green apples, avocado, fresh coconut

3) MEATS: Virtually all the meat including fish, poultry, and beef

4) VEGETABLES: Fresh, unblemed and freshly-crafted juice

5) BEVERAGES: distilled or filtered water, non-fruity herbal teas, stevia freshly squeezed carrot, stevia-sweetened, freshly squeezed carrot

5) FOUR THINGS:

6.VINEGAR

7) OIL: olive, grape, flaxseed, cold-pressed virgin coconut oil

8). NUTE: processed nuts, including pecans, almonds, walnuts, cashews, and pot seeds. Stored nuts appear to catch the mold, so look out!

9)SWEETENERS: stevia, Xylitol

10) DAIRY: biological chocolate, organic yogurt, cream cheese, unsweetened whipping cream (use the following in a sparing way), real sour cream.

Note: Again, such food choices are only allowed at the very start of the diet. After a while, you can introduce more and more foods, but only once the growth of the fungus is taken care of. He has built a few stages, so you're not left confused about what to do next. Remember that certain foods are limited only for a short period of time. I truly believe that if you continue your diet together with intermittent fasting, all the tools will be eliminated from fat loss. Losing weight is just eating more calories than you consume. Intermittent rapidity produces an immense calorie deficit, while the Phase 1 diet breaks down food addictions that cause overweight and fungal health problems.

Chapter Six:
How To Restore Your Diet From Abuse

You must be willing to stay on a diet for sufficient time to see results based on how much weight you need to lose. This could mean 10-12 weeks or even longer for real fat loss. To beginners as well as experienced dietitians, this is a difficult process; there is no trick or an easy way of reducing body fat other than low calories and a lot of exercises. A cheat meal once per week is a great strategy to help you stick to a program for a lasting, low calorie diet. After a diet ideally over the week, a 1-time meal of whatever you want (with managed portions) strengthens your body and does wonderful things in your mindset. Low calorie diets every day of the week can hunger the body and make weight loss more difficult. One healthy meal once a week with a lot of calories lets the body know it's not hungry, and it's okay to keep losing weight. A cheat meal once a week also helps to set an excellent objective every week, while also helping to manage food cravings. There is no question about the efficacy and rationale of using cheat meals once a week in your diet. There is a minor warning about cheat meals once a week...

This is the trick food lasting up to 6 hours. The leaner you get, the hungrier you get after a long diet. At some point, it becomes very difficult to control your appetite correctly in a meal of' anything you want.' Overeating or sometimes eating the wrong food mixture will put up to 6-10 lbs easily. Weight of scale. Depending on what you ate, it may take up to 4-6 days to remove, making your entire week of work just zero profit. When you use the cheat strategy once a week, try cheat meals (whatever you want) but only with very controlled portions. However, even after a strict procedure, you still find a cheat meal that fills your body with weight. For tips on how to recover / lose the fastest weight after a heavy cheat meal, please read the following paragraphs. Even if you do not actually have a strict regime, this method can still work well to clean the body after any food blowout.

Start your first morning with an intermittent quick after meal. Don't have your first meal until midnight, at least. Do not do so, if you are comfortable with eating as soon as you get up. Wait until noon to eat, at least. But get up several hours earlier and operate on a vacuous stomach. If there is time, the workout should be regular cardio plus a lightweight session. Plan to practice at least 1.5-2 hours prior to the first meal at 12 noon. The cardio you carry should be twice as much as you normally do. For example, if you normally walk on the treadmill for 30 minutes, you're 1 hour's walk. Then fill the rest of your 2 hours with more aerobic, calisthenic, and/or light weight lifting. Low enough poundages should be used to pump 10-20 reps with weight lifter. Don't lift vigorously and try thrashing the arm. Choose two exercises to add additional work to your body parts and/or to strengthen your weakness and override them for 4-5 sets of 10-20 reps. Finally, plan a hard cardio session at night (preferably about 6 hours later than the first workouts). Try filling as much cardiovascular and body weight as possible for an hour.

It should be sparse to eat the day after a cheat meal. A fast complete is not recommended, but a great dietary strategy; the intermittent rapid included is sufficient. Our aim this day is to eat very lightly and to stimulate bad food as fast as possible. Reduce the number of meals you eat this day first. When you eat only three meals normally, you can earn just two. You should have 3 plus a protein drink if you usually eat 5. Keep protein-rich with chicken, turkey, beef, lean red meat, eggs, and whey at least 25-40 grams per meal, which suits your lean body mass. Reduce your meals by eating more vegetables than starches even more on this day. If you only consume two meals, eat the carbs only with vegetables. Try to include at least 1 of your meals with a raw vegetable, such as large salads, raw broccoli, carrot sticks, etc. Keep fats at least on this day, too. Fats make your meals digest slower, and we want them to push you. If you need to make better use of the water, this is the day to do it. The day after a cheat meal, you want to drink as much water as possible to help to drive toxins and sugars through and to help improve digestion. On this day, do not drink any other drink than coffee and water.

You'll come back to your routine the next day (2 days after the cheat meal), just like nothing ever happened. You should be back on track by Wednesday or earlier after this eating / training plan (if your cheat meal was on Saturday). The results depend on how much damage the cheat meal has caused. The best results are obtained by keeping the cheat meal moderate first. It is also worth noting that this program, however, has not been tested on various subjects and can only work well for the author, who introduces the techniques and concepts. At the time of writing, the author had carried out a detailed bodybuilt diet routine of seven days / week, lifting weights 3-4 times / week for 1.5 + hours of sessions. If you are not in this process, how well this system will work for you is not understood. If it is not used to the amount of training mentioned above, the curriculum should be tailored to suit your individual needs and not tried to ensure that you are well enough without consulting a doctor.

What You Didn't Know About Weight Loss Diets That Burn Fat

You probably considered taking a strict diet if you want to begin a weight loss diet. This is good because the main part of weight loss is nutrition. You don't have to eat if you lose weight. What you have to do is to eat the right foods to encourage your body to burn excess fat on its own.

Now I'll mention some things you can eat so that your metabolic rate improves and all extra weight is burned.

Carbohydrates are misnamed by dietitians as they often find themselves in fatty foods and candies. Many people do not understand that carbohydrates play a crucial role in the growth of muscle tissue and have complex sugar chains. Because of this, the body needs a lot of energy to absorb carbohydrate-rich foods. You can naturally obtain carbohydrates from oatmeal, broccoli, and many other plants.

The advantage of complex carbohydrate foods is that they make you feel complete and thus avoid the risk of cravings. You won't have to suffer from hunger anymore, and a chocolate bar won't tempt you.

Another way to lose weight is to increase the consumption of your protein. As with carbohydrates, the body finds it harder to break down protein, thereby consuming more energy. Protein is also important in the creation of muscles. The more muscle you have, the more calories you consume while you are sitting at the office.

Ten quick weight loss diet tips for helping you get the most out of your weight loss program. There are many theories about the perfect way to lose weight quickly or the many tips and tricks on weight loss quickly. We are here to share some of the blatantly false claims, which teach you how to lose weight healthily.

The first thing you have to do is listen to the new research of a safe and effective diet and weight loss program that is not only endorsed by the' celebrities,' and that is tested and does not make you fat again, if and when your' will' power disappears.

Here are 10 of the most important things you need to know in your search for a loss of weight...

TIP #1: Don't get meals! Tip #1: If you skip a meal, it may seem to make sense to automatically lose those intakes of calories and thus help to lose weight... NO! Let me explain why not. Why not...

When you miss a meal, your brain reacts differently, and you're more susceptible to consuming and drawn to consume incorrect (fatty) foods than to healthy foods.

TIP 2: USE PLATES SMALLER! Yup! Yup! Sounds easy, or what? It has well proven that you are likely to eat up to 22 percent less food when people move from a 12-inch plate to a 10-inch plate! You should serve smaller portions on smaller plates so that your brain doesn't need to finish a large part. You don't have to eat, but just because it is there to eat!

TIP #3: WITH YOUR CALORY! Yes, I'm afraid you need to' count your calories' to effectively' diet' and lose weight! I can see that there are already many people heading for the next' miracle' drug, which will make you lose weight quickly. Hold on, and you'll have to learn a bit more about what you eat to lose weight successfully and maintain the' ideal' weight!

We all know that eating fatty foods will increase your heat and your weight will therefore rise, and you will be miserable longer than your pleasure! But you can also be forgiven for thinking you are healthy to eat when you're not... watch out for the hidden calories!

Tip #4: Don't improve your metabolism!: okay, then what if you are one of those people who seem to be eating the right food and to stay away from the unhealthy fatty lifestyle and still can't handle weight loss? Does your' slow metabolism' have to be right? Tests showed that: *Slow Metabolism Can Be A Myth And As Used As Excuse To Excuse Your Winne Excuse!* Do not be fooled by believing that your body has a slow metabolism as it is our brain, which is fooled by the fact that we do all we can to eat properly while ignored half the food we eat. However, portion size always counts if you eat healthily too, and our plate size can be drastic by that or cutting.

TIP #5: HUNGER PANGS PROTEIN STAVES! Okay, Okay on a diet to' stick to' or should I ask what you need to do to continue eating healthily? You don't have to get "starving hungry" basically! And here, you will discover that certain foods suppress the' hunger pangs' even more than others-demonstrated by the study.

So what kind of foods make you feel more comprehensive for a longer period? Protein... from every food group, eating a rich diet of protein might be the secret you need to help maintain hunger!

TIP #6: SUP KEEPS YOU SHALL FOR LONGER Is soup a reply? Could that be simple? Can soup in the diet be the "best-kept secret?" Essen food like a soup or a broth can dramatically impact our perception of hunger and the way the body translates what we eat into energy that is required for our everyday lives. Sure you may well have seen people praising the health benefits of smoothie, this simple and powerful method could have a significant impact on your hunger levels throughout the day and stop consuming more than you need in order to reduce the need for snacks between meals.

TIP #7: The Choice Weather, The Lord, you Are Eating! Tip #7: Buffets are bad for us! Buffets are bad for us! Yes, choice makes us who we are, but to have so much choice at a single meal makes us overeat or at least feels we miss the food we haven't tried! In fact, too much variety when choosing a meal leads us to over-eat; therefore, consider going on the' all-you-can-eat' buffet when considering a meal! Maybe you should also create a list of menus for the same calorie intake and adopt a fixed diet plan of foods to remove the' option factor!

Tip #8: Helps you to excrete more misery with LOW-FAT DAIRY! Milk, cheese, butter, and yogurt are generally one of the first things which people give up when they diet or at least decrease, based purely on the presumption that these products contain fat. Research shows that a higher diet of milk (calcium) helps the body absorb the fats even if you eat low calorie-fat healthy meals. In reality, they can help double the amount of fats that are excreted from the body! (I'm not going to go into the study details but take this as an inherent value study of real-life!)

TIP #9: EXERCISE GOES ON BURNING FAT, EVEN WHILE YOU SLEEP! Well, solutions for weight loss bears fruit like exercising more to help burn any unwanted fats stored in the body, but did you know you can burn off calories (and thus fat) during sleep? During exercise, our muscles use mainly carbohydrates to create energy because it is easier for the body to burn, and thus, after exercise, it takes up to 22 hours for your body to replace the carbohydrate. In the meantime, the body must find other outlets to burn off to at least maintain the basic functions alive! The body is actually forced to use fats to generate energy to keep you alive, walking, talking, and even sleeping!

TIP #10: WORKING AND LOSE! Well, exercise has its advantage when we help keep the excess weight and burn fat, but there might be an alternative for those who have no time (or inclination) to go to the gym... It makes sense just to keep moving and to be less' sedentary' that allows you to burn more calories and, therefore, fat. It's just small changes in our usual routine, which can help you lose weight. Try to look where you are more involved, leave the car in the shops or at least park away from the entrance to the supermarket parking lot! There are small steps which can have a big effect on your overall desire to lose weight and keep you safe and help you run out more calories in your daily routine, try to think less about how to really walk around and use calories.

Diet and women's fitness Methods

Weight is one of the most frequently discussed subjects today. 40% of adults in the United States alone are overweight, and 20% are considered obese. Diabetes, heart disease, high blood pressure, and cancer are some of the most common issues associated with overweight. There is an unprecedented number of children who become overweight and obese. This is partly because of their overweight parents ' bad eating habits. Parents should begin to lose weight now so that they can set a good example for their children.

Most of your advice on weight loss through the internet does not take into account that many people have busy lifestyles, and most advice is not aimed at many Americans on the go or advice to women. Most women's weight loss tips are focused on a diet and fail to consider the busy lifestyles that women work and come home and care for family and the limited time they have to cook a healthy meal. Several tips that women can use and incorporate in their busy schedules are provided here.

Many women know that they ought to cook healthy meals for their families every day, but the fact is that time isn't enough. A woman's busy schedule sometimes leads to late home and is too tired to cook. Some things you can do to make sure you have a healthy diet that doesn't bother you.

Eat Soup–Soup is a very nice and healthy meal, as it can be prepared with many healthy ingredients. When properly prepared, the soup will give you fewer calories and give you all the nutrients necessary to be healthy. In the broth, you should remove cream or milk. Use stock and water instead, which give it the same consistency without all calories. The good thing about preparing soup is you can do a lot, so all you have to do is heat it up when you come home.

Stop Carbon Protein Shakes-Do does not add carbohydrates and proteins. It will contain both too many calories and make it difficult to burn off. When you can't practice your time, this energy can simply become fat that remains in your body. Try to prevent a lot of carbohydrates and proteins from feeding at the same meal.

Eat Quick-You appear to "wolf off" your food several times when you are busy and take a short minute to eat it. We believe that our bodies say when we are finished, but in fact, it takes 20 minutes for our stomachs to tell our brain to stop feeding. If you eat too quickly, you risk eating too much that will create weight and eat food you don't want in your body. Slow down your diet, and your body loses weight.

Snacking–You hear a lot of snacking advice. This would work really well in an ideal world, but it doesn't actually work. You should not ignore your body when something is needed to eat, but the question is what to eat. If you need a snack, the best thing to snack is a fruit that will fill you and raise your strength. But drinking water is the best thing to do. It will fill you until the next meal, and it does not have any calories.

Chew gum-Chewing gum distracts you from hunger so that your body believes you eat. Do not underestimate the mind's power.

Friends exercise — It's very important to work with friends as friends will keep you motivated and hold you accountable to someone. If things start to get complicated, friends will drive each other. Even without this motivation, people tend to be discouraged and give up before they get the advantages of exercise. You shouldn't do exercise to feel like a chore. If you get into it, it can really be fun to practice.

Set goals-It is critical for you to sustain yourself to set realistic goals. When you set a goal, you must aim for something. Set yourself a time table so that you can manage all your activities throughout the day. Ensure that your goals are practical. If not, you're always going to be frustrated and think of leaving.

Set A Time To Exercise —For a busy woman, it is difficult to set aside time to go to the fitness center, so you must set up an hour or two for some kind of home fitness training. It's very important to find the time to practice. Even if you only start 15-20 minutes a day.

Know Your Limits-people are going to try to convince you how you should behave. Exercise in a way you feel relaxed. No one knows better your body than you do. Just do what you like and what you can do. If you like what you do, you will continue to do so, which in effect, will give you results.

Value your self-image-It's very important to consider what you're doing positive. Don't worry about what you look like when you're in the gym or jogging outside. Nobody judges you. The only thing people will have for you is admiration for having the same drive and determination to do something about your fitness and health.
So, try to follow at least some of these tips, and you will be slimmed down to your natural size soon.

Chapter Seven:
Women Need To Learn How To Do
The Right Exercises

Women must know how to do the right exercises because the male and female body reacts differently. In general, men can develop far more muscle mass than women can, but women can also achieve flat, but even ripped abs by doing workouts with exercises specifically designed for the female body.

You will simply learn how to relax your stomach muscles and even grow a slight six-pack. The following knowledge and training sessions for women show you the most effective and quick way to achieve this goal. You can use these exercises to get the flat stomach you always wanted but also to describe your muscles. As summer comes, you're going to look great in your swimming suit and short tops.

First, you want to continue your fitness with your training courses aimed at the lower muscles. The lower abdomen is smaller and weaker than other stomach muscle groups, so they are usually underdeveloped. This happens is that when you start your workout with the emphasis on the upper muscles, the lower muscles are exhausted and thus do not respond as you wish. Trying to get a flat stomach and ripped muscles would take far too much time to put the lower abs last.

Besides exercising for women, you must pay close attention to your diet. This now doesn't mean a trendy diet, a diet made up of high proteins or low carbohydrates, but a diet of balanced foods. Fresh fruits, whole grains, meat, essential fats, and healthy carbohydrates are recommended. Instead, consume six small meals instead of consuming three large meals a day, which will boost your metabolism in order to consume more calories.

It is also important that the intensity and speed of your workouts increase. If you want a fabulous belly, you can't do the same exercises at the same intensity all the time. Instead, you will manipulate the muscles with a range of exercises so that all different muscles can be used, and each exercise is amplified. It challenges the muscles to make the exercises more successful and to achieve the goal of a better stomach even quicker.

Ultimately, while you want a variety of exercises for women during workouts and you need to improve strength, you want to make sure that your muscles don't get overworked. You should never work more than four days a week, preferably three, to get the best results without reducing the risk of strain or injury and in the off days, concentrating on other core muscles while also cardiovascular work is important. Unfortunately, time and effort in your exercises are actually counterproductive when your muscles are overworked. With a few simple tips such as this, you will change your appearance and build stronger abdominal muscles that are good for your overall health. Although it might take a little more time to see the outcome you want, than if you were a kid, it would prove successful to be consistent with exercises and pick the most effective ones.

QUICK FITNESS TIPS FOR WOMEN

Is it something you want to be a fitness woman? Or is something you need to be more effective? Here are some fantastic diet and workout tips for women: 1. The most important thing is that each woman is different. Then think about looking for a program that best suits you. May software may not suit you since many women have a certain experience of surgery that should be taken into account. You should always consider consulting a certified fitness trainer to ensure that your fitness program does not cause adverse effects. Selecting the wrong software would only lead to injuries and disappointment.

2. Make sure the goals are practical. Fixing your mind to shape your body in a month's time would only increase frustration. You should ensure that the time you set is not unrealistic and that your body can achieve this. The software should be realistic and not

deceptive. One should be aware of their obstacles in everyday life so as to help achieve the efficiency of the program. After the program has been zeroed, you should set yourself a timeline and certain goals.

3. The exercises should focus on muscle-oriented body parts. This is because more calories are burned during muscle development and help to reduce fats. We suggest moderate weight lifting and multi-joint exercises. Multi-joint exercises save both time and effectiveness.

4. Muscle research should be carried out regularly. Your muscles should get harder over a certain period of time. It is not enough to lift the same weight with the same workouts and not to make the muscles work harder. The tracking of daily results will help you advance further by comparing it to previous data. Holding these documents helps build confidence because you can constantly check your accomplishments.

5. Exercises in a set of 10 repetitions should be carried out. The effort should be made to reduce the momentum for each repetition. This is because if there is less energy, the muscles must work harder. You can test your strength during exercise by seeing the movement of your head. The movement of the arm shows higher momentum.

6. One should make the exercise a little variety and flexible. A little change in the goals and activities every month helps to keep us focused and avoids boredom.

7. Motivation is the main thing!! Apprentices must pump up their energy levels, and the best way is to ensure healthy competition. Allowing trainees to have some influence allows them to be inspired because they know they are participating in the execution of the program.

Suppress Appetite Naturally

No, diet pills are the healthiest, most effective, and the safest method of avoiding and excessively consuming hunger binges. Over-eating is a very frequent problem that comes from the delay of food and is complete until your brain really realizes that and sends a signal to stop eating.

Here are some natural appetite management tips: eat as slowly as possible, and you are shocked that in the middle of the dinner, you no longer feel hungry and can easily avoid the habit of over-eating.

Eat a lot of frequent but small meals all day long. It decreases Appetite and avoids excessive consumption as soon as you start your next meal.

Have a lot of water with high fiber food. Fiber will easily make you feel full when you swell with water. Consider leafy vegetables such as cod, lettuce, and bokchoy.

Baked goods and sweets, as well as other refined sugars, should be avoided. Such kinds of "soft" foods are very high in calories and digested and consumed by our bodies very quickly and keep you hungry.

Try drinking a glass of water for at least eight glasses a day before each meal or snack and all day long.

These tips help you manage your Appetite naturally and reduce your hunger feeling. Nonetheless, bear in mind that hunger is a normal and necessary body reaction to tell us that it does not have enough calories to burn energy and now shifts to burn body fat. This is an integral aspect of weight loss, and natural appetite management is designed to reduce but not remove the feeling of hunger, as the diet would then be pointless.

It is easy because most people gain weight: they eat too much. It can be difficult to fight the urge to eat. Your hunger can be a mighty strength and impossible to resist. The good news is that you can actually put an end to your Appetite. In this chapter, I will share four of these tips and tricks to help you quickly lose weight. Let's begin... Let's start...

One of the main causes of extreme boredom is simple boredom. People who are bored frequently turn to food for their time. It's time for the things you love to do to fill your schedule. You will not only enjoy life more but will also find that you no longer feel hungry. It works just.

It's so easy that I'm surprised that more people don't hear about it. Eat More Protein You can quickly subdue your Appetite by increasing the amount of protein you consume. Protein helps you to feel more full for more time. It also has other useful weight-loss advantages. In your meal, I suggest that you include some protein. It will help you set the whole day.

It may appear counterproductive for weight loss, but it is indeed a powerful way to eat less. Eat more often. In other words, I mean calories. You have more food and snacks to eat, but they have to be small. Your overall calories must be lower than they currently are. You don't go hungry by feeding more often. You eat a little at a time, keep up and avoid feeding much on any single meal. Your Appetite is always regulated.

Drink More Water Let me stress that drinking water isn't a food substitute. I don't want anybody to go on a poor and unhealthy diet model. I just want to make sure you're not dehydrated. Not only is this unhealthy per se, but it often causes hunger, so that a water shortage will make you eat more calories your body really does not need. I suggest that you drink at least eight glasses of water every day, or more if the weather is warm.

In the end, you can do a lot to curb your Appetite naturally. Yet losing fat also means consistently exercising and eating healthy food. Therefore, become more involved and adopt a healthy food schedule for the best results.

Our food appetite leads to a lot of food and also a lot of weight. If this is allowed to take place all the time, certain health problems can arise if not avoided. The body only needs the right amount of food, and excessive eating can also cause various diseases and complications in the body.

It is sometimes very difficult to control our cravings with so much food and mouth-watering.

This problem has led people to discover natural appetite suppressants that work well with our bodies to control our food intake. Caralluma Burn, one of the leading appetite suppressants in the world today, does not focus as a dietary pill either to quickly lose weight but concentrates on how to get rid of food cravings.

As a result, someone who takes Caralluma Burn will experience a reduction in his Appetite and desire for food.

If you want a response to how your Appetite can be minimized, then Caralluma Burn is the best product you can take into account. This should also be part of your diet, along with a healthy exercise and the right amount of food to eat while taking Caralluma Burn. It is good to eat food with more protein intake than carbohydrates and fat-rich foods for quicker digestion. Eating a lot of fiber also encourages the body's water absorption, which makes us feel more healthy as well.

In combination with taking Caralluma Burn, these practices can lead to a faster and easier way of losing weight.

Deleting your Appetite can be a tough task that requires determination to succeed. With the use of these appetite suppressants, one can fight the Appetite for food, which is an impediment to an ideal weight.

Caralluma burn is a medium to prevent too much of one's eating. They include some suppressant that helps you balance the urge to eat plenty of food. The ingredient known as Caralluma Fimbriata extraction in Caralluma burn works in a way that reduces our hunger, which, in effect, prevents one from eating too much.

You can now enjoy and benefit from the advantages of a cleaner and more balanced body. You can get the body sculpture you always need by using Caralluma burn. Confidence and security have never been easy to live.

All you need to do is turn to a natural appetite suppressant drug, and you can guarantee a safer, more efficient way of life that will keep you always on top. If you are afraid to take risks in taking diet pills, you do not know about, try to invest in a natural and beautiful drug.

With Caralluma

Burn, you can guarantee that your Appetite can be suppressed automatically, so you won't have to worry about how to Suppress your Appetite.

The global slimming and consumer health industry continues to add new products to its portfolios. It would appear as if they are not without ideas, short of new ideas. Ideally, the choice between a man or a woman on the street and a celebration is natural slimming. The days of the risky but trendy pill for weight loss have ended. Why do you risk unnecessary health and well-being if natural slimming products compete with drug-based medicines? So much so that both the drug and the counter-market probably most effective diet medication is a cactus extract. Depressing Appetite is a consistent and commonly used strategy and has been used for decades. The reduction of Appetite is neither innovative nor the most effective natural way to reduce body weight, reduce a Body Mass Index, and promote healthy loss of weight over the long term.

The main theory behind suppressing Appetite is not to eat as much as you would normally during the typical day. The practice is not much harder to do. The one major factor that increases our weight is that we can not control what we eat. When our belly gets used to expect a certain amount of food-the need and urge grows even more over time.

It is our brain that craves food that ultimately causes our problem when it comes to gain weight. It's our brain that craves food. It's the brain responsible. A part of the brain is known as the hypothalamus. While having to delve into mechanics too much, the hypothalamus controls how the body feels when it comes to blood pressure, temperature, and hunger.

Occasionally, our brain doesn't want food, and it's a snack. Our brain will send a message to our body that it is not actually food. Water is the easiest and most efficient way to stop Appetite. This is a message that weight loss manufacturers or anyone with a monetary interest in the food industry are too willing to spread.

The best-known suppressant drug is Hoodia Gordonii, a plant like a cactus growing in the Kalahari Dessert's arid plains. The natives of this region had not always afforded the luxury of water and thus found it possible to survive days without the need for food or water when consuming part of the Hoodia Gordonii plant. Hoodias can quench thirst and hunger. Although it is not advised to go for days without water-conditions often dictate. Tribesman of the Kalahari had lived for centuries with Hoodia plant and was their best-kept secret until ten years ago when the western world discovered their national wealth.

Nowadays, Hoodia is sold worldwide, and the consumer has access to patches for dozens if not hundreds of diet pills marked Hoodia.

If you want to incorporate Hoodia carefully into your health research, Hoodia quickly becomes a diet pill to be replicated by the market.

A Powerful Tool For Weight Loss & Diabetes: Intermittent Fasting

First and foremost, fasting is not hunger. Hunger is the involuntary abstinence from eating induced by external forces; it occurs in times of war and starvation when food is scarce. Fasting is voluntary, deliberate, and regulated, on the other hand. Foods are readily available, but for social, environmental, or other purposes, we choose not to consume them.

Fasting is as old as humanity, far older than any other diet. Ancient civilizations, like the Romans, understood the inherent value of intermittent fasting. These have often been referred to as cycles of treatment, purification, or detoxification. Almost every culture and religion on earth perform certain fasting rituals.

Due to agriculture, people only eat three meals a day, plus snacks. We only eat when we found a food that could be isolated hours or days. From an evolutionary point of view, eating three meals a day is not a survival condition. We wouldn't have survived as a species otherwise.

We have all forgotten this ancient practice before the 21st century. Fasting is really bad for business, after all! Food producers allow us to eat multiple meals and snacks a day. Nutritional authorities caution against the serious health consequences of missing a single meal. Such signals have been drilled in our minds over time.

Fasting doesn't have a regular length. It can be done for several hours to several days to months. Continuous fasting is a diet routine in which we switch from fasting to normal feeding. In general, shorter fasts of 16-20 hours are done more often, even daily. Longer fasts are usually done 2-3 days a week, 24-36 hours a day. As it happens, between dinner and breakfast, we all easily spend 12 hours each day.

Millions and millions of people have been fasting for thousands of years. Is it unhygienic? No. No. In fact, numerous studies have shown that the health benefits are enormous.

If we eat regularly, what happens?

Until taking advantage of intermittent fasting, it is best to understand why it is unhealthy to eat 5 to 6 dishes every day or every few hours (exactly the opposite of fasting).

When we feed, we eat food. Insulin (produced through the pancreas) is the main hormone involved, which rises during meals. Both carbohydrates and protein stimulate insulin. Food causes a minor effect of Insulin, but the food is rarely eaten on its own.

Insulin has two main functions-First; it allows the body to start using food energy instantly. Carbohydrates rapidly become glucose, increasing blood sugar levels
— insulin channels glucose into the body cells for energy use.
Proteins are divided into amino acids, and excess amino acids can become glucose. Protein does not necessarily increase blood glucose, but Insulin can be increased. Fats have a limited insulin effect.
Secondly, insulin stores excess energy away for future use. Insulin converts excess glucose into glycogen and stores it in your liver — however, the amount of glycogen that can be stored small. When the limit is reached, glucose is fat in the liver. The fat is then placed into the liver (overly fatty liver) or into fat deposits (often stored as visceral or belly fat) into the body.

So when we feed and snack all day long, we are constantly fed, and the amount of Insulin remains high. It means that we can spend most of the day storing food energy.

Which happens when we quickly?

The cycle of using and storing food energy when we eat goes backward when we fast. The level of insulin drops, and the body begins to burn saved energy. Glycogen is first accessed and used as glucose that is stored in the liver. The body then begins to break down stored body fat for energy.

The body exists therefore in two states—
the fed state with high Insulin and the fasting state with low Insulin. Either we store energy for food, or we burn energy for food. When food and fasting are matched, there is no increase in weight. If we eat and store energy the majority of the day, there is a good chance that over time will become more important.

The portion-control strategy to consistently minimize calories is the most common dietary guideline for weight loss and type 2 diabetes. The Diabetes Association, for example, suggests an energy deficit of 400–650 kcal/day paired regular physical exercise. Dietitians observe this method and prescribe 4-6 small meals all day long.

Does the portion control strategy work on a long-term basis? Rarely. Rarely. A cohort study of 176,495 obese patients with a 9-year United Kingdom follow-up revealed that only 3,528 were able to achieve normal body weight by the end of the study. This is a 98% failure rate!

Intermittent fasting is not a constant restriction of calories. Restricting calories causes hunger and worse compensatory growth, a decrease in body metabolic rate, double curse! Because it is more difficult to lose weight as we eat fewer calories a day, and much easier to get back into weight after we have lost it. This kind of diet puts the body in a "hunger mode," as metabolism reverses for energy retention.

Intermittent fasting has no such inconvenience.

Health benefits of intermittent fasting Increase weight and body fat loss metabolism Unlike a daily diet for calories, intermittent fasting increases metabolism. From a survival point of view, this makes sense. When we don't feed, the body uses stored energy as fuel to keep us alive to find another meal. The body's hormones cause energy sources to be transferred from food to body fat.

Research clearly demonstrates this phenomenon. For example, the Basal Metabolic Rate increased by 12 percent over four days of continuous fasting. Norepinephrine, which prepares the body for action, increased in neurotransmitter levels by 117 percent. Blood fatty acids increased more than 370 percent when the body switched from fuel to stored fats.

No loss of muscle mass Unlike a constant calorie diet, intermittent fasting doesn't burn as many people fear. Throughout 2010, researchers looked at a group of subjects who had simultaneous fasting for 70 days (one day and the next day). Their weight started at 52.0 kg and finished at 51.9 kg. In other words, there was no loss of muscles, but 11.4 percent was lost in fat, and LDL cholesterol and triglyceride levels improved significantly.

The body produces more human growth hormones naturally during fasting to protect magnetic muscles and bones. Normally, muscle mass is maintained until fat falls below 4%. Many people are, therefore, not prone to muscle wear when they do intermittent fasting.

Type 2 diabetes is a disorder in which the cells actually have too much sugar in the body, to the point of the cells no longer being able to respond to Insulin and consume any more blood glucose (insulin resistance), resulting in high blood sugar. The liver is also loaded with fat, while it attempts to clear the excess glucose and turn it into protein.

Therefore two things must happen to reverse this condition-first, stop putting more sugar in the body.

Second, burn off the remainder of the sugar.

The best diet to do this is a low-carbon, medium-protein, and high-health diet of fat, even ketogenic. (Remember that carbohydrate most raises blood sugar, some protein, and some fat) This is why a low carbohydrate diet can help reduce incoming glucose burden. This is already sufficient for some people to resist Insulin and type 2 diabetes. In more severe cases, however, diet alone is not enough.

What about the workout? Exercise helps to burn off glycolysis, but not all tissues and organs, including the fatty liver, in skeleton muscles. Certainly, exercise is important, but it is necessary to temporarily "starve" cells, to remove excess glucose in the brain.

This can be achieved by intermittent fasting. That is why people have historically named regeneration or detox fasting. It can be a powerful tool for removing all excesses. It is the fastest way for blood glucose and insulin levels to be reduced, and insulin resistance, type 2 diabetes, and fatty liver to reverse.

By the way, Insulin for type 2 diabetes does not address the root cause of the body's excess sugar. Insulin can indeed lead to lower blood glucose from the blood, but where is the sugar? The liver will only make it all fat, fat in the liver, and fat in the abdomen. Patients who take Insulin usually get more weight, which exacerbates their diabetes.

Improve heart health Overtime, high type 2 blood glucose can damage the heart vessels and nerves. The longer you have diabetes, the higher the risk of developing heart disease.

The risk of cardiovascular disease and stroke is also decreased by rising blood sugar by irregular rapidity.

Brainpower boosts.

Multiple studies found that quicking has many neurological benefits, including attention and focus, reaction time, instant memory, awareness, and new brain cell development. Mice studies have also shown Intermittent quicking reduces inflammation of the brain and prevents Alzheimer's symptoms.

We normally feel starvation about four hours after a meal. What is to be expected with intermittent hunger? So if we easily last 24 hours, does it mean that our feelings of hunger are six times higher? Of course not. Of course not.

Most people worry that fasting would lead to extreme hunger and unhealthy food. Research has shown that the day after a strong day, there is generally a 20% rise in caloric intake. Nevertheless, hunger and appetite decrease unexpectedly with prolonged fasting.

Hunger is coming in waves.

If we do nothing after a while, hunger dissipates. Taking tea (all sorts) or coffee (with or without caffeine) is often sufficient to combat it. However, it is best to drink black if a tea cubicle or two or half creams does not react much to insulin. Do not use sugar or artificial sweeteners of any kind. Bone broth can also be taken during fasting if necessary.

Blood sugar does not crash

Sometimes people worry about blood sugar falling very low during fasting and getting shaky and sweaty. This actually doesn't happen because the body closely monitors blood sugar, and multiple mechanisms are available to keep it in the correct range. The body begins to break down glycogen in the liver during fasting to release glucose. It occurs during our sleep every night.

If we quickly last longer than 24-36 hours, glycogen stores are depleted, and the liver produces new glucose with glycerol, a by-product of the fat disintegration (a gluconeogenetic process). The brain cells can also use ketones for energy, apart from the use of glucose. Ketones are produced when fat is metabolized, and up to 75% (25% from glucose) of the brain's energy consumption is supplied.

The only exception is diabetic and insulin-treated people. You Should consult your doctor first, as the dosages would possibly have to be may when you fast. Otherwise, you have to have some sugar to counteract it if you are overmedicating and if hypoglycemia occurs, which can be harmful. It breaks up quickly and makes it counterproductive.

The dawn phenomenon
Some people experience high blood glucose after a period of fasting, especially in the morning.

This morning activity is the result of a circadian rhythm that instantly precipitates a higher level of several hormones to prepare for the next day
- adrenaline-to provide the body with energy.
- Growth hormone—to help in the regeneration and production of new protein
- Glucagon, transferring glucose from storage in the liver to the blood as energy.

The frequency of blood sugar rises in non-diabetics is low and not even considered by most people. Nevertheless, a significant blood glucose spike may occur for most diabetes as the liver dumps sugar into the blood.

This will also occur in long fasts. If there is no food, the level of insulin remains low, while the liver releases some of its stored sugar and fat. It's normal and not bad at all. When the liver is less filled with sugar and fat, the frequency of the spike decreases.

Who shouldn't fast intermittently?
- Women who want to become pregnant, pregnant, or breastfeeding.
- Those who are underweight or malnourished.

- Kids under 18 and parents. kids under 18.
- Those who gout. Those who gout.
- Gastroesophageal reflux (GERD) disease.
- Those with eating disorders would contact their physicians first.
- Diabetic medications and insulin need to be checked with physicians first as dosages need to be every.
- Those who take drugs should contact their physicians first, as the duration of the prescriptions can be influenced.
- Those with high stress or problems with cortisol should not be rapid because it's another stressor to easy.
- Those who train hard most days of the week shouldn't be fast.

How to plan for intermittent quickly?

It is best to transition to low-carbon hydrogen, high-healthy fat diet for three weeks if anyone is thinking of starting intermittent fasting. It allows the body to get used to using fat instead of glucose as an energy source. This means removing all sugars, grains (bread, cookies, pasta, rice) and vegetable oils. This will eliminate the most fasting side effects.

For example, start with the shortest space of 16 hours, from dinner (8 pm) to lunch (12 pm) the following day. You will normally eat two or three meals from 12 p.m. to 8 p.m. Once you are confident, you can prolong it easily to 18, 20 hours.

For shorter fasts, you can do it continuously every day. You can do it 1-3 times a week for longer fasts, such as 24-36 hours, alternating between fasting and normal days of feeding.

There's no perfect fasting scheme. Choosing one that works best for you is important. Many people get results with shorter speeds; others may need longer speeds. Many people do it quickly; some do tea and coffee quickly; others do a bone broth quickly. Regardless of what you do, staying hydrated, and controlling yourself is very necessary. You can stop immediately if you feel ill at any point. You may be thirsty, but don't feel sick.

Conclusion

In the past, food programs for women were merely a decrease during portion sizes. The large dining plate is replaced by the bread plate. The serving sizes have been reduced accordingly-and so the waistline height!

Life is not so simple nowadays, and diets for women have to be individualized to answer a number of questions that affect the way we live right now. In this short chapter, I put together women based on standard lifestyles and suggested dieting strategies for women that matched these categories.

First and foremost, this is a diet just like me for women! The working mother has a constant risk of constantly consuming processed food and prepared meals and refined foods as well as feeding to meet the demands of irregular meals. At the outset, a healthy food plan for the working mother should be planned. While creating fat loss programs for women with a career, I usually encourage them to add those evenings, lunch, and snack foods to their regular shopping list. It includes an extra loaf of bread, additional greens, and more cheese. Although the majority of women's weight loss plans concentrate on a wider choice, there is nothing more boring than consuming the very same salad and cheese sandwich for snacks when it is a takeaway food or an easy warm snack that you can purchase. Switch food every week. Every week. It's easy to have breakfast, toast, fruit, and yogurt. Again, when the package runs dry, swap the cereal. With respect to the evening meal: use the oldest female strategy weight loss plan in the book: decrease your plate size! Mom: you're too busy to worry about single meals! Eat the same thing: just try to eat a lot less.

The weight reduction scheme for women below 30 can be enormous and exciting without babies! You have plenty of time to eat and delicious food! You're lucky! Start every day with a smoothie juice based on organic, fat natural yogurt, and fruit! Shop for fruit yogurt and add fresh fruit again! Your entire body will be energized, and all calories will be consumed! Try eating new delicacies with a minimal dressing of salads. Go to a coffee shop every day and buy a fresh green salad. Try asking them to wear goat and olives and add the balsamic dressing. Make sure the salad is big and also have fresh bread in size! This weight loss diet includes dinners that are not made of carbohydrates for women under 30. Only stay away from beans, spuds, and bread. It will make you hungry around 9 am and make you stretch for chocolate. Take some time to eat organic beef, chicken, and fish, along with many good veges. This girls diet program is simple, enjoyable, not precise-and yet works. Enjoy your food while you can!

The last women's weight loss program is for women over 40 years old. I'm all girls with you! It's pretty simple for you. Weight is more difficult to change. You're going to have to do a lot of physical exercises. Forget about thirty minutes, three days a week. For at least one hour, four or five days a week, you need to work hard. Without this, no female diet program can show good results. In addition, you will adhere to either of the above listed fat loss programs for women-as you may also be a working mother with children. If you're lucky enough to be part of a stage of your life, follow the menus for women under 30 but fit with your evening meal into a small portion of carbohydrate. I am talking about half a prepared cup of rice or half a baked spud. Be alert; excessive carbs make you hungry later—hurrying up for the biscuit jar at 9 pm!

I sincerely hope that these three women's eating plans are straightforward: yet they are effective. Don't fuss. Don't fuss. Just try and hit the gym, walkways, bicycles, and roads as much as you can! Good dieting! Happy dieting!

Printed in Great Britain
by Amazon

55391634R00208